## Praise for *How to Heal Yourself W*

"Amy Scher is a voice of calm, reassuring wisdom. Her own triumph over illness is truly inspirational, but what really puts Amy in an inspirational category of her own is her warm, kind, down-to-earth, truly accessible approach … This book is a must-read for all who are dealing with health challenges, but also for everyone who wants to shed old blockages and free themselves to experience their very best health and live their fullest, most authentic lives."

—Sara DiVello, bestselling author of *Where in the OM Am I?*

"Amy's story is awe-inspiring. Her book *How to Heal Yourself When No One Else Can* is full of wisdom and easy-to-implement techniques that have the power to help anyone reconnect their mind with their body and their heart with their soul and heal their entire lives. A really beautiful read."

—Luminita D. Saviuc, founder of PurposeFairy.com and author of *15 Things You Should Give Up to Be Happy*

"Amy Scher's *How to Heal Yourself When No One Else Can* is a comprehensive and user-friendly DIY manifesto that's the real deal. Amy guides readers toward authentic self-healing in a way that's easily accessible, honest, and relevant for today."

—Chris Grosso, author of *Indie Spiritualist* and *Everything Mind*

"Amy is a courageous pioneer in the field of mind-body-spirit healing. She has created a practical, compassionate, and intelligent book that empowers you to heal and improve your health. With proven, easy-to-follow techniques, you will gain insight into the root cause of pain, physical dysfunction, and illness and transform your health … This book illuminates the path to wellness."

—Sherrie Dillard, author of *Develop Your Medical Intuition*

"In this refreshingly honest and approachable book, Amy Scher offers practical tools and step-by-step guidance to help you 'hear' what your body is trying to tell you, clear unprocessed emotional baggage, and enhance your intuitive abilities. This is a how-to guide for anyone seeking a deeper, more peaceful connection with their body, mind, and spirit—and a happier life."

—Jordan Bach, life coach and founder of TheBachBook.com

"An inspirational story of one woman's quest to overcome a life-threatening disease. Ms. Scher proves once again that self-knowledge and the courage to be one's self are the foundation of healing and good health…This is a must-read for anyone ready and willing to heal themselves on the levels of body, soul, and spirit."

—Keith Sherwood, author of *Energy Healing for Women*

*How to*
# Heal
# Yourself
*When No One
Else Can*

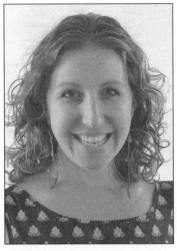

© Craig Vershaw

## About the Author

Amy B. Scher is a leading voice in the field of mind-body-spirit healing. As an energy therapist, Scher uses energy therapy techniques to help those experiencing illness and those in need of emotional healing. She has been featured on healthcare blogs, CNN, *Curve* magazine, *Elephant Journal*, and the *San Francisco Book Review*. Scher was also named one of *The Advocate*'s "40 Under 40" for 2013. She lives in California and can be found online at AmyBScher.com.

# How to
# Heal
# Yourself
# When No One
# Else Can

\* \* \* \* \* \* \* \* \* \* \* \* \* \* \*

**A Total Self-Healing Approach for Mind, Body, and Spirit**

\* \* \* \* \* \* \* \*

## AMY B. SCHER

Llewellyn Publications
Woodbury, Minnesota

FIRST EDITION
Tenth Printing, 2022

Cover art: iStockphoto.com/41606416/©embra
iStockphoto.com/16357774/©Vectorig
iStockphoto.com/9457829/©Vectorig
Cover design: Ellen Lawson
Interior illustrations: Mary Ann Zapalac, except the Healing Tree on page 234 by
Llewellyn Art Department

Llewellyn is a registered trademark of Llewellyn Worldwide Ltd.

Library of Congress Cataloging-in-Publication Data

Names: Scher, Amy B.
Title: How to heal yourself when no one else can : a total self-healing
approach for mind, body, and spirit / by Amy B. Scher.
Description: Woodbury, Minnesota : Llewellyn Worldwide, [2016] | Includes
bibliographical references and index. | Description based on print version
record and CIP data provided by publisher; resource not viewed.
Identifiers: LCCN 2015043634 (print) | LCCN 2015039069 (ebook) | ISBN
9780738747286 () | ISBN 9780738745541
Subjects: LCSH: Energy medicine. | Mind and body therapies. | Healing. |
Self-care, Health.
Classification: LCC RZ421 (print) | LCC RZ421 .S34 2016 (ebook) | DDC
615.8/51—dc23
LC record available at http://lccn.loc.gov/2015043634

Llewellyn Worldwide Ltd. does not participate in, endorse, or have any authority or responsibility concerning private business transactions between our authors and the public.

All mail addressed to the author is forwarded but the publisher cannot, unless specifically instructed by the author, give out an address or phone number.

Any Internet references contained in this work are current at publication time, but the publisher cannot guarantee that a specific location will continue to be maintained. Please refer to the publisher's website for links to authors' websites and other sources.

Llewellyn Publications
A Division of Llewellyn Worldwide Ltd.
2143 Wooddale Drive
Woodbury, MN 55125-2989
www.llewellyn.com

Printed in the United States of America

## Other Books by Amy B. Scher

*Lessons from Lyme Disease, Chronic Fatigue, and Fibromyalgia:*
*A Collection of Stories, Insights, and Healing Solutions*
(2014)

*This Is How I Save My Life: From California to India, a True Story Of*
*Finding Everything When You Are Willing To Try Anything*
(2013)

*Llewellyn's Complete Book of Mindful Living: Awareness & Meditation*
*Practices for Living in the Present Moment* (contributor)
(Llewellyn Publications, 2016)

*For my clients, who are the bravest bunch I know.*
*These words are all for you.*

# Acknowledgments

To Charlotte Phillips, my wife, my best friend, and my person. You are the biggest, most incredible surprise of my life, and proof that the universe knows exactly what it's doing. Thank you for always being the "wind at my back" and never "the spit in my face." You graciously love me through all my moments and there isn't anyone I'd rather love back. You and me against the world, baby.

Thank you from the bottom of my overflowing heart to my family: the Fockers (on both coasts and in the UK). There are no words that accurately describe our clan, our crazy, our love. Your support and entertainment are something I don't know how I got lucky enough to have. You are a tribe that I never want to be unglued from.

To my MB (mama bear), Ellen Scher: Thank you for editing until your eyes boycotted, and then editing even more. But mostly, thank you for your unconditional everything. Our late-night phone calls in hysterics over some very questionable typos made for moments that exist only in a whirlwind of mother-daughter love. You are my hero.

There is no adequate way to thank Steve Harris, my literary agent, my friend, and half of the coveted Team 22. I remember emailing you once to ask if you'd still be my agent even if our project didn't sell. I didn't have to wait five minutes for your reply: "You are my author 'til death do us part (or until you don't want me no more)." I waited for you almost my entire life and you did not disappoint. Thank you for being all I ever dreamed of in an agent. Thank you for being honest when my writing was "too boring" to show editors. Ha! You were right. You're always right. And thank you for also being one hell of a cool lunch date.

I offer my deepest gratitude to the team at Llewellyn, particularly Angela Wix, my editor, who saw something special in me among a very crowded world of authors. I can't thank you enough for your kindness and patience and for helping me to get to the freakin' point just a little bit faster. Where were you my whole life? You are simply, literally, the best. And to Andrea Neff, a massive thanks to you for your exquisite talent, focus, brilliant insight, and attention to detail. You helped me to make this book even better than I imagined.

Immense gratitude to the following individuals who, because of their contributions, made this book possible. Melissa Gentzle: you've always believed in me more than I do, and it never goes unnoticed. You are a cheerleader like no other, and you're gonna be an amazing mama for it. Julia Montijo: who edited sample chapters into the wee hours even though you had your own "big girl job" to do, and also for teaching me that when you grow up, you get to make the rules. Cheers, my love! Amanda McAulay: who made me eat lunch and gave me pep talks unconditionally. Thank you for embracing my crazy and being a truly wonderful friend. Nadine Nettman Semerau: we are the only two left in our writers club, but we have proved it was well worth hanging in there. I still can't believe the crazy awesomeness that has unfolded for us and I can't wait to stick together for more. The 84th Street neighborhood crew: you edited, organized dinners, and kept my life real when I was stuck at my desk. You are the best neighbors two girls could ask for. TMW: thank you for being the very best listener I know, and for having my twin brain so I never have to explain anything but you still always know what I mean. Dale Paula Teplitz: thank you for changing everything I ever believed about teachers. You are absolutely exceptional. Kate Kerr Clemenson: thank you for flying halfway around the world to save the day when I needed it the most, and for sticking around when you realized what you were in for. Reality check accomplished. Sara DiVello: my "partner-in-writing-crime." I can't thank you enough for the phone calls (ohmygosh, the phone calls) and for the countless number of times you had to say, "Seriously, you've got this." And for the times you also said, repeatedly, "Yes, really. You do." You've made me believe in instantaneous friendship. I hope we write many more books together and always have each other's literary backs.

I can't go without sharing my never-ending gratitude for the insatiable Shannon Sheridan. How can I thank you for planting those seeds so many moons ago, way before I was ready to water them? This book only bloomed because of you.

And finally, thank you to my circle of angels on the other side. You know what you've done.

# Contents

# Exercises and Techniques

These are the exercises and techniques that you will learn throughout the book. The five main techniques are indicated with an asterisk.*

### Chapter 7

To clear unprocessed experiences:

### Chapter 8

To release beliefs:

### Chapter 9

To transform unhealthy patterns:

### Chapter 10

To repattern the fear response:

### Chapter 11

To have a guide for your healing journey:

# Images

## Disclaimer

The publisher and the author assume no liability for any injuries caused to the reader that may result from the reader's use of content contained in this publication and recommend common sense when contemplating the practices described in the work.

\* \* \* \* \* \* \* \* \* \* \* \* \* \* \*

# How to Rock This Journey

Imagine you are a beautiful, sprawling tree. You have a big, strong trunk, roots that stretch deep into the earth, and branches that reach toward the sky. One day, you notice something isn't quite right. Your leaves are brittle and full of little holes, and your branches are drooping with heaviness. Upon inspection, you can't find any obvious reason for this change in your state of being. You start to panic immediately and take better care of your leaves and branches. You spray them and medicate them and more, but nothing changes. The leaves you are working with are merely the visual result of whatever the problem is with your tree.

The soil of this tree represents your foundation. The soil is where it all comes from. It's who you really are at the core. It's the sum of all the things that have influenced you. All the rocks and rubbish that have gotten mixed right in with you will affect every part of the tree. Everything in that soil becomes part of your being.

The roots of your tree represent the energy system and pathways. If your soil is full of imbalances—just as a tree's soil could be full of environmental stressors—those roots will become imbalanced from your soil, too, and affect your entire beautiful tree. It may take some time for its effect to reach your leaves and branches, maybe even years. But eventually it will.

The leaves of your tree represent your organs, glands, muscles, body systems, chemicals, and hormones. By the time you find those little holes in your brittle leaves, you will not be able to bring the tree back to health by treating the leaves directly. You can't just spray the problem away. True healing will not come from caring for your leaves in retrospect. It comes from going deep into your soil and correcting the base from which the tree grows. You have to come back to who you really are by clearing away those old energies that are contaminating your base. You just have to clean up that soil.

## How This Book Will Help You

The biggest stumbling block to harnessing our own self-healing power is knowing what to address—in other words, knowing *how* to heal. This is true whether you feel emotionally imbalanced or those imbalances have affected your physical body, too.

The process I am going to guide you through in this book will show you *how* to heal. You will learn how to clean up your soil following a model that has been successful for myself and hundreds of others, through the client sessions I've conducted. You don't need to be sick to use this book. In fact, this book is not about illness; it's about emotions and energy. And those are two things that each and every person can benefit from balancing for a greater sense of well-being. Remember, cleaning up your soil is the end game, your only goal. And cleaning up that soil can change your life.

While there are countless energy therapy techniques out there today, many require another person to act as an aide for your healing. In this book, you'll learn some of the self-application techniques I used in my own healing. Some will be ones that I learned during my journey, and some will be ones I created. All of these techniques will give you full power over your journey. You will not need to depend on another person to help you perform or practice any of them. It's all in your hands, baby!

You'll learn several main techniques for changing your relationship with stress:

- Thymus Test and Tap
- Emotional Freedom Technique (EFT)
- The Sweep

- Chakra Tapping
- 3 Hearts Method

Outside of the main techniques, you will also be learning others that will help carry you on your journey. You can find a complete list of all the exercises and techniques in the front of this book. When I teach you the techniques, there will always be explicit instructions. That's the only way I can communicate the ideas to you. If you see the instructions as merely suggestions, though, you'll get so much more from them. If you feel called to do something a slightly different way, then do so. It's likely it will work for you better that way. I personally tweaked and put the "Amy twist" on every technique I learned. If you want to do this too, you have my permission to go wild. The types of deviations I made to techniques during my own healing included things like using my right hand instead of my left hand, holding a pose or technique for a longer or shorter period of time than stipulated, skipping a certain part of an exercise, and more. All of these alterations are okay. There isn't a single technique I use with my clients or myself that is exactly how it was taught to me.

No matter what techniques you use to clear energy blockages, always know that finding *what* to clear is more important than what energy technique is used for the actual clearing. That's what we'll be discovering together in different ways throughout this book. This will be the most effective approach and will give you freedom from worrying about doing each technique perfectly. Once you know what to clear, you are free to integrate any energy healing techniques you currently use into the various aspects of healing.

## How to Use This Book

This book has been written in part as an exploratory process, in part as a how-to, and the rest as stories, insights, and examples to keep your soul full while your healing is happening. The examples I share are from real sessions in which my clients volunteered and/or gave me permission to tell their stories. Even so, each client's name and identifying details have been changed completely to fully protect their privacy.

Many of the stories you'll read are from my time in India, which taught me lifetimes of lessons, and I intend to pass them along to you for your own journey. I have outlined lots of different things you can explore to help you lead a happier, more fulfilled and peaceful life in a content body. It may feel like there is a lot for you to work through, and maybe there is. But it *can* be done, and there is no time limit. Tread gently, my friend. Be easy on yourself.

The most effective way to understand my approach is to read, learn, and practice what I share in the order it's presented, from start to finish. It's the best way to absorb the big picture, concepts, and techniques. By the time you have finished the book in its entirety, you will have deep knowledge of my approach, and may then continue your work by going back to any parts of this book in any order you wish. In addition to reading and practicing at your own pace, I invite you to find others interested in doing this work so you can support each other along the way. When I was healing, I did it completely alone and often wished I had a group of like-minded people to share and discuss all my new discoveries with. That's why, at the back of this book, I've provided a list of book club discussion questions. I encourage you to find a tribe, talk about what you're learning, hold each other's hands, and make healing a team effort. Whether you do this alone or with a group, embrace the guidance that resonates with you, fully into your life. Make it a part of who you are and use it to make what you already have richer. This book shouldn't be treated like a to-do list. Let your brain adjust to the concepts and keep your heart open as you allow things to process. You will likely find you are led to things not even outlined here. When you get that nudge, it's your intuition and the universe whispering, "Follow me." Just know it's safe to go.

The main concepts of this book are laid out in parts:

- *Part One: Surrender, Accept, and Flow.* This will cover the importance of learning to be okay where you are in your journey. You will learn why it's essential to surrender, how to do so, and how it can catapult your healing forward. From within the space of surrender, you have an opportunity to lay a beautiful groundwork for your healing. This will include simple shifts in energy and thinking patterns that will strengthen your foundation to support what is to come.

- *Part Two: Identify Blockages*. This part will discuss exactly how to identify blockages through the use of muscle testing and learning the language of your body. You will be guided into learning exactly what you need to clear for your complete healing.

- *Part Three: Change Your Relationship with Stress*. This part will explain what stress is and how your internal reactions to stress can be transformed in order to help you heal. It offers detailed instruction on exactly how to do that. For each of the techniques I teach you, I'll offer suggestions to help you apply it directly to your own specific situation.

Once you've covered each of the chapters in this book, you'll essentially be going through all of these parts simultaneously during your healing. It is not a step-by-step process in which you need to go in perfect order and check each part off the list before moving on. Instead, this healing process is much like cooking a four-course meal. You don't necessarily do one thing at a time, seeing it through to completion, and then start the next. The goal is for all of your steps to eventually manifest as a dish that you love (yourself!), but to make that happen, you are constantly stirring, turning, and attending to several things over and over.

There is no rush or clock set for you. Instead, set the intention to create something beautiful and the universe will expand the container in which you'll have to explore and grow.

In chapter 11, I'll offer you a detailed illustration of the Healing Tree—an overview of the entire process you've learned. The Healing Tree illustration is a virtual map of *you*, the beautiful tree we talked about earlier. It is a snapshot that summarizes the four main areas of imbalance that you'll learn about in this book, and the techniques to address them. I've placed the illustration at the very end of the book because it will be your best companion, but only once you've learned all the working pieces that go into it. You will then be able to step back and see its usefulness as your own personal guide map.

## Where Should You Begin?

At first, in my own journey, I was determined to release all my "problems" in a systematic, pragmatic way. I tried to create a nice, neat formula to organize the way this healing journey would unfold. The good news is that it doesn't work like that. The even better news is that you most definitely don't have to attain perfect balance or release *all* your stuff in order to be well. Phew! The body does not need to be stress- or problem-free to attain deep and complete well-being.

If you're feeling like you'll never get better unless you do it all and get perfect and get every little thing in order, here's the answer to your worries: YOU DON'T HAVE TO FIX IT ALL. YOU DON'T HAVE TO FIX IT ALL. YOU DON'T HAVE TO FIX IT ALL. I still sometimes have emotional meltdowns, my body hurts temporarily, and I find imbalances and blocks in my energy system…but I'm happy and well. You can heal without doing everything. You can heal by just making a dent. YOU DON'T HAVE TO FIX IT ALL.

Clients often come to me and say, "I have so many problems. Where will you start?" And I say, "Don't worry, you really only have three to five core issues and everything else is likely connected to those." Everything is so interconnected that, while focusing on one imbalance, we may also be unknowingly correcting others.

For example, I was once helping a client with persistent digestive problems. She was experiencing acid reflux, nausea, and bloating with pretty much everything she ate. While our focus remained primarily on the goal of repairing her digestion, she got a very welcome surprise. After a few sessions, she noticed that in addition to her digestive symptoms improving, her phobia of speaking on the phone (something she hadn't even mentioned to me) had improved as well. Because one issue can be connected to many others, we are often doing more extensive clearing than we realize.

That experience is a perfect example of why we shouldn't get caught up in doing things too methodically. We need only remember that the goal of becoming who we really are is the finish line. It isn't some attaining of perfection, balance, or even always a physical healing. It's just to release all that prevents us from living freely. It doesn't matter how you get there; it just matters that you do.

Healing is really just practicing. Each day of your life you have an opportunity to practice letting go of what keeps you from moving forward and closer to yourself. When it seems like it's working, keep practicing. When it seems like it's not, keep practicing.

## What to Expect

While using the techniques in this book, you may feel immense relief immediately or it may require great persistence. Either one is fine. It has no bearing on your ultimate healing.

When moving energy, there is always some "processing" that occurs—meaning your body is releasing that energy completely from your field, which extends far beyond your physical body. During this process, which can last a few days to about a week, you may feel an increase in discomfort, fatigued, or a little bit uneasy. An equal number of my clients feel lighter and better after sessions though, so that is highly possible, too. As you're moving and clearing energy more consistently, you'll become attuned to your body's release process. If you feel you are having a difficult time with processing, I've provided some tools in chapter 12 that will help you.

While using these techniques, you might find your mind wandering. That's a natural occurrence and is nothing to be concerned about. Often the mind is wandering to things that are somehow related to what you're clearing. And even if not, no harm will be done. As you perform the techniques, you might yawn, burp, get the chills, have a runny nose or eyes, cough, feel emotions strongly, hear your stomach gurgling, sweat, or experience any number of sensations. All of these things are good indicators that your body is releasing. This means that it's coming out of stress mode and moving into relaxation and healing mode. Specifically, yawning signals that your nervous system is relaxing. I have a number of clients who experience no signs of energy releasing during the process and benefit greatly anyway. When I am moving energy, whether for myself or with a client, I yawn a lot. If it's something really big, I tend to sneeze. I always joke that one sneeze is worth ten yawns for me! Sneezing and yawning are my own body's responses to shifting a lot of energy, but each person is different and you'll get to know your signs, too.

It's equally important to remember that we all release energy at different speeds. I've done so many sessions where my client immediately feels better from the work. I call these "one-session wonders." Almost instantly they see symptoms shift or feel a huge emotional relief. This is definitely not my pattern, though, and it may not be yours either. If for some reason you don't feel anything at first, it may just not be your body's pace, or there may be many more layers to work on.

If your challenge has been long-standing, it might take a while of working at it from different angles to feel a shift. Your challenges did not show up overnight, even though that's how it might have seemed. They were brewing in your energy system long before they manifested as symptoms that you paid attention to. The good news is that healing often works like this too. Nothing's happening, nothing's happening, nothing's happening (you think)... and then, all that was happening inside suddenly shows up for you to see! Your healing could be right around the corner at any given time. Seeing the journey as an integrative flowing, weaving uncovering of your life is the most fulfilling and effective way to approach it. For deep and permanent healing, there is no quick fix. You have to surrender and let it all unfold. The universe doesn't give "no's," but it does sometimes give "not yet's." Just keep showing up and doing what you need to do. Healing never happens fast enough for us, but that doesn't mean it's not happening.

During my own healing, I didn't keep meticulous track of what I was working on or how it was going; I just made sure to *keep going.* Most of the time I had no idea what I was doing, but I dedicated myself and I consistently used what I learned. It was a winning approach for me. If you consistently use the techniques, you will win too.

I suggest that you keep a notebook, casually jotting down whatever comes to you during your own journey. While symptom-tracking and record-keeping of every past hurt and emotion will not be helpful here, it can be useful to have a place to write down ideas that you have, subtle shifts you see in your symptoms, and observations you become aware of along the way.

## How Much Time Should I Dedicate to the Process?

Imagine a pot of vigorously boiling water with a lid on it. Eventually the water gathers so much steam that it bursts though the lid and overflows. You run to the rescue, lift the lid, and release some of the pressure. But you don't then walk away and come back a week later. You tend to the water. You keep letting a little steam out in between doing other things in the kitchen. While you too can release "steam" (energy) from your body by doing deep work now and then with the techniques you learn in this book, it will be much more effective if you consistently release the pressure a little bit at a time. Keep on top of it. Dedicate time daily. It doesn't have to be hours. Sometimes working on certain things will take longer. However, becoming frozen and doing nothing because you "don't have time" or are overwhelmed is perhaps the biggest mistake I see.

Sometimes clients will tell me at the start of a session that they've had a really hard time with something in between our working together. "What technique did you use to move through it?" I always inquire excitedly. Sometimes they reply, "Oh, I didn't do anything." That's when I try not to cry myself! Feeling bad is a grand opportunity to clear whatever is coming up and just begging to be released.

If you are feeling strong emotion even outside of the time you've dedicated to your healing, use a technique to release that "steam" in the moment, lest it get added to the pot that you'll have to tend to later. If you are feeling sad or jealous, have an upset stomach, or whatever it may be, use the moment to figure out what's coming up for you (I've provided lots of ideas for this in chapter 6), and apply a technique that you've learned. Did you have a bad dream last night? Use that as an opportunity to find something to clear. Are you still stirring over something that happened at work last week? Deal with it. All of this is coming up because it has deeper roots that can be gently cleaned out.

Five minutes, ten minutes, or however many minutes you have on a consistent basis can change your life. With this book, you will have the tools you need to do it. The techniques are gentle and effective. They work. As always, it's all unfolding and happening in divine time. It doesn't need to push or rush. All is well. You *are* healing.

## Important Chapters to Reference

While each chapter in this book is important, there are a few in particular that you will want to reference often. I'd like to point them out here so you can quickly flip back and forth.

- List of Exercises and Techniques following the table of contents—Here you will find a list of all the techniques and exercises that are in this book. This will allow you to flip quickly to where you need to go.

- Chapter 6: Learn the Language of Your Body—This chapter can be used as a kind of reference guide and will give you a deep understanding of what your body is saying to you through its symptoms. Each and every time your body appears to be malfunctioning is an opportunity to see it in a different light. Your body will be a great guide in your healing.

- Chapter 7: Clear Unprocessed Experiences and Chapter 8: Release Harmful Beliefs—These two chapters present four of the main techniques that you will be using. For each, you'll learn how to use it, apply it to your challenge, and see examples of how that's done. Note: the fifth main technique is taught in chapter 9.

- Chapter 11: Create Your Unique Map for Healing—This chapter offers a snapshot review of everything you learned throughout the entire book. It includes an illustration of the Healing Tree to help you visualize the process, along with directions on how to use the illustration to streamline your healing.

You are now ready to get started. My parting words to you are short but important: Persistence and patience are not always natural virtues. The miracles they deliver, though, absolutely work and are definitely worth it. And so are you.

# An Introduction
# to the Energy Body
# and Self-Healing

*Chapter One*

\* \* \* \* \* \* \* \* \* \* \* \* \* \* \*

# My Success Story

*It's only when caterpillarness is done that one becomes a butterfly… You cannot rip away the caterpillarness. The whole trip occurs in an unfolding process of which we have no control.*
—RAM DASS, *BE HERE NOW*

I wasn't doing anything noble at age twenty-five, like changing the world, but I *was* totally content making people smile with "Live To Ride" Harley-Davidson paraphernalia and meditating to the sound of rumbling bikes on my lunch break. In July of 2005, I had no idea that my dream life as a marketing director for Harley-Davidson was suddenly about to fold, although I see now that I had ignored many warnings of deteriorating health that came in the years before. At first I began having trouble walking up the gentle ramp from my office at Harley to the community kitchen. I had pain and tingling in my legs. Shortly after that I started to lose function of my arms. My dexterity slipped away, I couldn't lift my arms above my head to wash my own hair, and I tripped and fell more times than I could count. Doctors were puzzled, I was terrified, and my neurologist ordered me not to return to work.

I was in pain twenty-four-hours a day, with relief only when I was in a drug-induced sound sleep. Fierce, full-fledged body pain engulfed my being. There was not one inch of me saved; everything from my feet to the top of my head was screaming in agony. Because the disease was misdiagnosed and untreated for so long, the damage to my body was ravenous. Exposed nerves in all my limbs created firing pain with no rhythmic pattern to warn me when the worst was to come. Full-blown arthritis in my major joints left me unable to lift my leg high enough to step over the bathtub and into the shower. I often could not even sit on the toilet without assistance because my hips could not handle the pressure of lowering my body weight to the seat. I couldn't use my shoulders to push myself up on the bed to get out of it when I wanted. The lining of my heart became inflamed, leaving it constantly racing as if I had just run a marathon. I was so fatigued that I could not move my lips to speak at times, and I had cognitive impairment so compromising that I couldn't form words to get them to my lips anyway. A severely weakened immune system made me a host for recurring shingles so severe that they scarred and hurt for years afterward. My white blood cell counts plummeted so much that I was unable to leave the house at my immunologist's insistence. No organ or system in my body was spared. My life as I knew it was swallowed away and replaced by a monstrous disease that any doctor had yet to understand. I was almost more terrified of living than dying.

## Trying to Heal

Several years after a string of misdiagnoses and treatments that nearly killed me, I was finally accurately diagnosed. This is the jackpot moment in a chronically ill person's life. Apparently, a tiny tick bit me, doctors explained—a tick that I had never even known about. It transferred to me bacteria called *Borrelia burgdorferi*, the causative agent of Lyme disease. Lyme disease is a bacterial infection transmitted from a tick bite that can cause serious health problems if left untreated. And it did. The diagnosis of Lyme disease carried with it a string of further diagnoses, including autoimmune thyroid disease, kidney dysfunction, connective tissue disease, fibromyalgia, neuropathy, and more. I never had a visible bite, rash, or anything of the sort. I had been tested for Lyme disease before, but the testing for Lyme is so flawed and did not deliver a positive result until many years too late, when my blood was sent to a specialty lab. I took my late-stage Lyme disease diagnosis like an oversized bag of groceries at the checkout stand; I wrapped my arms around it as best I could, and I moved on to find a cure.

The Centers for Disease Control and Prevention (CDC) estimates that approximately 300,000 cases of Lyme disease are contracted in the United States annually—with a mere 10 percent being properly diagnosed.[1] That estimate makes Lyme disease twice as common as breast cancer and six times more common than HIV/AIDS. Some cases are never even reported. This leaves many with misdiagnoses such as fibromyalgia, lupus, chronic fatigue syndrome, multiple sclerosis, arthritis, migraines, learning disabilities, bipolar disorders, Parkinson's disease, heart arrhythmias, and more.

Despite heavy-duty antibiotic therapy to try to eradicate the Lyme bacteria and other co-infections that were transmitted by the tick, I was still in a constant state of suffering. Alongside my very intensive protocol of forty-four pills and intramuscular antibiotic shots every day, I had exhausted the gamut of alternative possibilities. While I was functional enough to be without constant care by the time I found out about Dr. Geeta Shroff, the founder of a stem cell clinic in Delhi, India, I still had a slightly less severe form of all of my symptoms. My Internet research on Dr. Shroff revealed very mixed opinions about her, from "hero" to "con artist." But after talks on the phone with Dr. Shroff and following other embryonic stem cell patient's stories, I knew the stem cells had the potential not only to boost my immune system but also to regenerate damaged organs, nerves, and cells in my body. It felt like this was precisely the dose of kick-ass that could save my life.

On December 9, 2007, just nine short months after the Lyme disease diagnosis, I boarded a plane for New Delhi, not knowing if the treatment would save my life or kill me. Catapulted into a country that swept me off my feet in love and constantly tested my sanity at the same time, I knew my heart needed both of those things equally. With as much grace as I could muster, I aimed to embrace it all, including

---

1. "CDC Provides Estimate of Americans Diagnosed with Lyme Disease Each Year," Centers for Disease Control and Prevention, August 19, 2013, www.cdc.gov/media/releases/2013/p0819-lyme-disease.html.

copious amounts of curry, rambunctious monkeys everywhere, and fear that flooded every inch of me.

While my die-hard optimism had always served me well, it quickly became apparent that it would not satisfy the requirements of a culture that promotes "mind over matter," "think positive," and other concepts that caused me to blame myself for my illness. "The stem cells can do their part, but you have the power to heal yourself," Dr. Shroff repeated almost daily, like a broken record I was trying desperately to stop.

After nine weeks of daily stem cell injections and enough personal growth opportunities for a lifetime, I left the clinic walking on my own. The success did not come easy, but it came. With a struggle that I can only compare to wrestling an elephant to the ground, I was cured. Or so it seemed.

## The Return of Symptoms

It was a couple of years later when I experienced the initial ripples of a healthquake on what had felt like stable ground for some time. During a two-month trip to London, I found myself with disturbing pain and tingling in my feet that seemed to appear out of nowhere. Weeks went by and it persisted. By the time I sought medical help, things had gotten so bad that I was admitted to the hospital for two days of testing. MRI and other diagnostics came back negative and I was released. The familiarity was haunting though—these were the exact symptoms that had appeared in 2005 at the beginning of my career as a full-time sick person. While I did test positive for the Epstein-Barr virus, food allergies, and a host of other items pointing to immune dysfunction (again), there were no positive indications of Lyme disease.

It seemed that all at once, unruly forces inside of me were colliding, culminating in an all-too-familiar "here we go again" storm. But as suddenly and mysteriously as the symptoms appeared, they faded just as fast, with no treatment whatsoever. However, my near-lifetime struggle with endometriosis, fibroids, polyps, and intensely painful menstruation became increasingly worse. Each month brought days on the couch with prescription narcotics in an attempt to dull the pain. Many times, though, the medications wouldn't even take the edge off and I would end up in the hospital. None of the four surgeries prior to my stem cell treatment, or the one after, provided relief for longer than a few months' time.

Overwhelmed by being in London and trying to find a doctor familiar with Lyme disease, menstrual issues, and the cocktail of other diagnoses from my past, I decided to follow a new lead. During one of my marathon Internet searches, I stumbled upon a Traditional Chinese Medicine doctor who, I read, had seen Princess Diana as a patient. During my first appointment with the sweet but not overly chatty doctor, I stared at Princess Di's picture on her bookcase. *Anyone who could help the princess could surely help me*, I determined, immediately feeling a new sense of security.

Traditional Chinese Medicine (TCM) is an ancient medical system that is thousands of years old. It is built on the foundation that symptoms arise from blocked energy in the body's subtle energy system. When those imbalances are corrected using different modalities, a healthy flow of the body's energy is restored.

Every couple of weeks, I went for acupuncture and was sent home to drink offensively bitter tea that made my kitchen in London smell like a rotting tree. In time, I did in fact see some marked improvement in my pain, energy levels, and particularly my premenstrual symptoms. Sadly, though, when I became lackadaisical about my ritual of boiling, sifting, and hesitantly choking the tea down my throat, my improvement slowed drastically. I suspected I needed more time to see the long-term benefit, but the costly and physically nauseating treatment plan soon became too much to manage.

By the end of the year, I was back home in California, feeling like all of my options had slowly drained away, like water from a cracked bucket. I began again the process of reaching out to specialists and getting lost in the chaos of medical decision-making. Then, from somewhere in my brain (probably stored in a folder labeled "Come Back to One Day"), Dr. Shroff's words bubbled back to the surface of my consciousness: "You have the power to heal yourself." And just like that, I decided I would try.

How could a radical treatment like embryonic stem cell therapy save my life but not my uterus? Why were my menstrual cycles getting worse? Why were some of the food allergies and other ailments from before stem cell therapy resurfacing? What in the world was the cause of that episodic pain and tingling in my legs, and would it be back?

I was not sure yet why all of this was happening, but I knew I was getting closer to something—and I threw my faith toward the idea that the very something I needed was just around the corner.

### Discovering Energy Work

Perhaps I was headed in the right direction with addressing my body's energy system, but had not quite arrived at a solution yet. I longed for a process that didn't include dependency on long-term appointments or boiling, sifting, draining, and plugging my nose as part of the treatment protocol. I started to research other types of therapy that addressed the body's subtle energy system.

When I eventually came across the term *energy medicine*, I was drawn to it immediately. Energy medicine is a process of balancing and enhancing the energies of your body for well-being. I read everything I could about it, being particularly glued to the works of Donna Eden, a pioneer in the field. I bought all of Donna's books, starting with *Energy Medicine*, and began to practice several energy medicine techniques each day. Eventually I started to see some improvement. I noticed the painkillers I had been taking for fifteen years during my menstrual cycle were actually helping now. Before, they did little if anything. Something intangible felt different, too. I felt sturdier, perhaps even a tiny bit happier. I sensed that I was solidly on the right track.

I thought this was *it*—the thing I'd been waiting for—until I realized my oh-so-limited attention span was not conducive to "babying" my energy flow. In between menstrual cycles, I'd spend an hour or more each day making sure my energy wasn't getting stuck. During menstruation, I had to be attentive to it at all times, doing exercise after exercise to lessen the pain. My new job of constantly monitoring this natural womanly process (that I despised so much) was counterintuitive.

Despite feeling like I hadn't quite figured it all out yet, I continued to follow some of Donna's energy medicine protocols but made a decision to deepen my healing approach. I wanted to learn why or how my energy was getting stuck in the first place.

Why do some people heal permanently and completely while others don't? I had met several people during my journey who were cured from their ailments by what seemed to me like a stab of simplicity in my back—vitamin B shots, quinine supplements, eliminating gluten, or similar easy fixes. Why not me?

I quickly came to an epiphany: *If treating the body alone doesn't resolve the problem, then maybe the body alone isn't what caused it.*

## The Missing Pieces to Positive Thinking

While I had always considered myself to be an eternal optimist, I had started to think I was a school-of-positive-thinking failure. Or maybe it was just a bit more complicated and I hadn't gone quite far enough yet. What if the profound effect of thoughts and emotions was so massive that it was the entire basis of my failed health?

That's when I began gently looking at my life—not with fault or blame, but from this heart-shaped hole inside of me that felt like it was waiting for just this moment, a knowing that I had some filling up to do. I became open to the possibility that my life, and myself, had contributed to where I was, even if it didn't make complete sense yet. After all, I was the common denominator in a pattern that seemed to manifest in different illnesses at several different times in my life.

Clearer than I'd ever seen anything, I suddenly became aware of my deficiency in the art of letting go, in being vulnerable, and in trusting life. I always tried to control everything in life, for I was convinced my world would be safer that way. I have always had to remind myself to breathe during times of stress; otherwise I would naturally hold my breath. I often fought back tears when they wanted to flow, wanting to be the type of person affected by nothing. My emotions felt safer in the confines of my body, and I never considered the cost.

My mind is logical, calm, and collected, and I often treated my heart as if it should be the same. I have always been "the rock," as many of my friends call me. I instinctively felt that taking on everyone's problems was my plight in life, and I accepted that plight without thought.

I thought I had flawed intuition, but I began to realize that I ignored it when it whispered to me. I was uncomfortable with making decisions based on anything but justifiable data—I am a Virgo to the core. I allowed myself to need logic and legitimate reasons to free myself from relationships that weren't good for me, career paths that didn't fit me, and more. And, I was run by fear—not the kind of fear that shows up in phobias, but the kind of fear that made me feel unsafe every day, in every way.

I read. I researched. I sat. I absorbed the works of Dr. Bernie Siegel, Louise Hay, Dr. Bruce Lipton, Caroline Myss, Wayne Dyer, Gary E. Schwartz, Candace Pert, Masaru Emoto, and other experts. I became cognizant of the possible implications of what I was discovering—that unprocessed emotional energy, unresolved experiences, limiting beliefs about how the world should work, fear, negativity, and generally allowing yourself to be separated from what was in line with your heart … could make you not only miserable but sick. It was the missing piece of the positive-thinking puzzle for me. While "think positive!" had gotten me far, it fell short of turning the tides of my life toward complete healing.

All of these newly realized pieces contributed to burdening stresses that I now believe were weighing just too heavy, even for a body virtually reborn after stem cell therapy. Looking back, I am absolutely sure that the fear of a Lyme relapse was so imminent that it itself contributed to the degradation of my health again. I believe the "all clear" from my doctors in London was enough to coax my body out of internal panic mode and back into healing mode. But I knew that having an awareness of this fear mode was just not enough. I needed to find a way to transform the pattern if I wanted to be, and stay, well.

## You Have the Power to Heal Yourself

I think it was clear to Dr. Shroff that I may not have had the capacity to believe her words at the time, but she knew I was close.

I finally stopped. I just stopped. I stopped pointing to symptoms and syndromes, and the perceived external causes of those. I turned within instead. There is a saying that when the student is ready, the teacher will appear. How true it is. The information that I discovered was not brand-new, just like many of our "realizations" or "epiphanies" do not often come from information we've never encountered or that isn't already held within us. The key is readiness. You can see or hear the same thing a hundred times, but not until you are ready will your whole self receive it. I needed to get to a point of being so finished with the disease, the burden, and the struggle that I just refused to participate in it anymore—not in a way that caused me to fight it or be angry at it, but in a way where my spirit was truly done. I was ready to take a deep breath, surrender to a new starting point, and complete the experience I had been going through.

Suddenly, I was able to recognize the times in my life when I had been complacent about being sick, perhaps believing at a subconscious level that it was my way out of carrying everyone else's weight. Giving myself permission to take care of me first was an unfamiliar ability, but one that came easily with illness. Maybe I even believed at some level that being sick afforded me a level of safety I couldn't conceive of otherwise. It sheltered me from a world in which I found it too hard simply to be comfortable with being myself. With all of this, I separated from my own inner being and strayed off course, apparently so far that my body was talking to me in the only way it knew how—through symptoms.

The process of self-discovery and releasing all that no longer served the life I so desperately wanted was not dramatic or earth-shattering, but it was life-or-death important. Using a three-part approach that I'm going to share with you in this book, I did what doctors couldn't do for me, what stem cells couldn't do for me, and what many said would never happen: I healed completely and permanently. There is one thing I became absolutely sure of in the process of it all. It was not the bacteria alone that caused the Lyme disease and it was not solely a hormonal imbalance that caused my menstrual issues. I believe that the stem cell therapy ignited the physical repair of my body. This was undoubtedly supported by personal growth during my time in India. But eventually the impact of going back to life as usual caused the subtle erosion of my health again. I changed my physical body, but I did not change my life and my relationship with it. Not only do I know that emotional imbalance dramatically affected my immune system, but I believe my body was trying desperately to get my attention too. It was trying to tell me that the way I was living my life wasn't in line with the *me* I was meant to be. I learned about the possibility of remanifesting illness if one fails to address the origin of it.

Playwright Katori Hall described it best when she said, "It was like God was holding a bag of blessings and I was holding a bag of shit, and when I let go of my bag, God was like, 'Here you go.'"

I was just ready and it was just time. I didn't care about excuses anymore or the details of how I got where I was. I was not attached to my story or blaming the bacteria, virus, or hormones that were taking me down. I was simply willing to see that if I was part of this challenge, I, too, was part of the solution.

To this day, people still ask me, "How did you know how to heal?" And the truth of the matter is that I didn't. But I was ready to do my part to try. Being sick was not my fault, but if I wanted to get better, it had to be my responsibility.

I squeezed my eyes tight and let things unfold instead of forcing my way through. It took a colossal amount of bravery to turn in this direction, but it is possible for anyone to do. I decided I had no choice left but to trust so deeply in where I was being led that if I were to fail, I could still be nothing but proud of myself. I both embraced the journey and let it go from my hands, a balance that perhaps tops my list of life's greatest achievements. I participated in my life's path while still allowing it to unfold in its own way and time. When I made this mental shift, everything became easier. I slowly opened myself up to exactly what I needed to do, at just the right time it needed to be done. I allowed something to come through me and trust a process that was greater than myself.

Your path, too, will unfold in its own perfect timing, revealing pieces of the puzzle only as they are ready to be healed. It will not always be in *your* time, but it *will* happen. The challenge is to show up and do the work, knowing that what you want is already making its way to you.

In each moment that I was overcome by fear and doubt, I focused on those simple words of Ram Dass: *Be here now.* And when I got through that moment, I did it again. I sometimes stumbled along, but I continued to learn new ways to access my energy system, and if it resonated with me, I applied it.

Whatever did not resonate, I left behind. I ventured far beyond positive *thinking* and aimed for something even higher: positive *feeling.* I did this by diving right into the deep dark unknown of myself, uncovering things that no longer worked for me—beliefs, energies, emotions, and patterns. And through much trial and error, tears and triumphs, I healed myself to my very core using nothing but my own internal guide. I wasn't perfect, not by a long shot, but I did what I could, as often as I could do it. And it was enough. Little by little, I dropped my bag of shit, and as I did, the blessings came. The allergies faded, the Epstein-Barr virus retreated, and my immune system built itself back up as a strong and abundant force that cannot be easily shaken.

## Becoming the True You

Everything about well-being sits firmly on this very simple rule I've learned: You must become who you really are. You must be the real you. That means to love, accept, and be yourself no matter what. You can't contract your energy for others, or for fear, or for anything else. No light-dimming or living small allowed. This journey of healing is to be yourself. In fact, true healing is not measured by reaching a place where you are free of negative emotions or have even attained a physical healing. I truly believe that straying from and separating from your inner being, or who you really are, is the root of discontent in the mind and body. You are not broken and do not need fixing. You are not wrong and do not need righting. You are not in need of self-help; you are in need of self-love. The only thing you need to do is find yourself, and stay there.

There are many ways in which we diminish our true selves. It is easy for me to say, "Be the true you," or "Become who you really are," but it can be difficult to recognize how we are *not* doing or being that. As we grow into adults, we can drift so far from our true nature that we lose our reference point for who that person inside really is. In an effort to conceptualize this idea for you, I am offering you my own very personal list as an example. These are the things that I now see caused me to suppress my truest, deepest light—and, subsequently, contributed to illness. I suggest you make a similar list of all the ways you think you are doing the same. You might be as scared making your list as I am sharing mine, but we are all born brave.

- **Fear**—I called it "anxiety" my whole life and never resonated with feeling "scared," but I was fearful deep down in my bones. Here are *some* of the things I was scared of: fear of sharing and expressing emotion, fear of failing at anything, fear of people being upset with me, fear of trusting myself, fear of my parents dying, fear of getting in an accident or being hurt, fear of getting injured in sports, fear of making a mistake, fear of travel and small spaces, fear of crowds, fear of germs, fear of not being in control of everything, fear of not having money, fear of people disapproving of me, and the list goes on. We are most definitely not meant to live dominated by fear.

- **Relationships**—I found myself in relationships I knew weren't right for me. The relationships themselves created situations where I would avoid speaking up and would incessantly worry about upsetting my partner, feel as if I wasn't interesting or fun enough, and hold myself responsible for fixing my partner's insecurities. Perhaps even more damaging, I wasn't honest with myself about these relationships. I talked myself out of what my intuition was saying—that the relationship wasn't healthy for me. Talking ourselves into anything that's not true in our gut causes inner conflict and is harmful to our being. All of this tailoring and filtering of myself prevented me from being me.

- **Challenging Myself**—While in some ways I took too much responsibility for things, in other ways I copped out. From the time I started working, I rarely had jobs that felt good. I never enjoyed school or felt good at it, so I shut myself off from pursuing education that could have helped me find something enjoyable. I was so full of self-doubt about school and didn't even try to go to a four-year college because I was terrified to take the required testing. I essentially limited the choices for my life because I was *scared of a test*. This is the silly stuff we do. I do not in any way believe that someone must have a college education to be successful (I still don't have a degree and am totally content with that), but I do believe we must call ourselves to our greatness. We need to hold ourselves accountable to do hard things. We can't shy away from scary things that would help us move forward.

- **Self-Criticism**—I was terribly hard on myself. In fact, if it had been someone else, it would have been considered abuse. I beat myself up over every little mistake and imperfection and always expected more of myself than was humanly possible. I had difficulty being able to just let go and have fun without constant monitoring of my behavior. Joy is part of our true nature, and suppressing it is extremely counterintuitive to well-being. Learning to be easier on myself was not only beneficial, but absolutely necessary.

- **Self-Sacrifice**—I had an intense opposition to hurting people's feelings, even if it was unintentional. Because of that, I avoided it at all costs and I paid the price, emotionally and physically. I did things that I didn't want to do, I put myself last, I never said no to others and yes to myself, I made sure I suffered *for* someone if I could spare them, and I was far too understanding of people who hurt me. Self-sacrifice shows up in many ways and is always detrimental.

I hope this list gives you some solid examples of how we block our true selves from coming forth. When I share it with clients, they often say things like, "Wow, I can't imagine you could be that screwed up!" I laugh because I know there must be things missing from that list. But

I am most definitely proof that one can come out of all of this on the other side, happier and healthy.

The most important thing is to move through it all and find a way to be unapologetically you. The more you can do that, the better your life will feel. It's called being "in alignment" (with who you are, not with everyone else), and it's more amazing than you can imagine. Your energy will flow, your body will be in full healing mode, and you'll be on your way to miracles. As a bonus, life will also be super fun and a million times easier than it is now.

The biggest work of our lives is releasing anything that does not fit within that paradigm. It doesn't always happen overnight, but as long as you are willing to "be here now" over and over again, I can say with complete honesty that this work is for you.

In fact, I live my life as an example to you of being healed—a combination of living a spiritual life in a body that feels good while also sometimes eating too much pizza, losing complete Zen-like perspective, and practicing being a beautiful human mess. This journey of true and lasting healing is not one that cuts you off from the world and reality. It's one that integrates the best parts of you right into it all. "The big question," as Joseph Campbell says in *The Power of Myth*, "is whether you are going to be able to say a hearty yes to your adventure."

Now, are you ready to drop your bag of shit and take the coolest trip of your life?

*Chapter Two*

\* \* \* \* \* \* \* \* \* \* \* \* \* \* \*

# My Approach to
# Mind-Body-Spirit Healing

*Being yourself is hard. Living with the regret of having lived your*
*life according to other people's expectations is hard. Pick your hard.*
—JORDAN BACH

When I was diagnosed with late-stage Lyme disease in 2007, I was shoved into a whole new world. It seemed the common consensus among patients was that even doctors couldn't fix *this*. Growing up, I knew doctors only as heroes and my personal safety net. When we were sick, we'd go to them and they'd fix us. So now again, they would come through, I was sure. But after torturous years of failed medical treatments, I was finally faced with the truth: sometimes even a hero is gonna have to let you down.

It was then, and then only, that I ever even entertained the possibility that there was another way this all worked besides a simple equation of *physical ailment equals physical fix*. It turns out, there is way more to it than that.

In this chapter, you'll discover the basics of the energy body, how certain kinds of stress affect the energy body, the importance of self-healing, and my three-part approach to healing. This will give you a strong foundation of understanding for what you'll experience with this book.

## The Body's Energy System

Our bodies are so much more than what we see. Actually, everything is so much more than what we see. Everything is really just energy.

Let's take a quick trip down memory lane to elementary school science where we most likely learned, and then forgot, that everything in the universe vibrates. Each and every atom has a specific vibratory motion. Each motion has a frequency (the number of oscillations per second) that can be measured in hertz. Frequency, simply put, is the rate of electrical energy flow that is constant between any two points.

Just as the universe operates on energy, we as human beings operate on an intricate energy system too, one that affects all of our organs, muscles, glands, and more. It is fueled by electrical impulses that run through us.

This energy system is at the core of how our brain functions, how our muscles and nerves receive messages from the brain, and how our moods and thoughts interplay in our lives. You may already be familiar with the concept of energy in the body because of the use of EEGs measuring brain waves, EKGs measuring the electrical activity of the heart, and other diagnostic medical tools. Much energy in the body can be easily measured with tools like these, while some energy, often referred to as "subtle," is not yet detectable by these types of tools. Some types of subtle energies include electromagnetic energy, magnetic vibrations, and biomagnetic fields. Subtle energy is something that has been seen and felt by healers and energy-sensitive people for thousands of years.

Many ancient medical systems, including Traditional Chinese Medicine and Ayurveda, are based on the body's energy system. Within the energy system of the body there are various types of energy patterns, like chakras, meridians, auras, layers, and more. The two patterns we will be working directly with through techniques in this book are meridians and chakras. Meridians are energy pathways in the body. Each meridian flows through the body, delivering energy to the organs and tissues along its designated pathway. You'll learn more about meridians in chapter 7 when you learn Emotional Freedom Technique (EFT). Chakras are spinning energy centers in the body that hold old stories. Each chakra governs a specific part of the body and affects the organs and tissues in that area of the body. You'll learn more about chakras in chapter 8 when you learn the Chakra Tapping technique.

When our energy fields are being disrupted, flow irregularly, or become sluggish and blocked, we can begin to experience symptoms. Energy disruptions can be felt in the body. They can feel like there is a knot in the pit of your stomach when you're scared, burning in your chest when you're hurt emotionally, or an achiness in your back or neck when you're in a state of inner conflict. You are experiencing what happens when your energy isn't flowing properly to your organs, glands, and muscles with the energy they need to thrive.

Energy flows through different areas in our bodies. If there is a blockage in one part of the energy system, it will likely affect some of the other organs, muscles, and glands connected by the same energy flow. For example, the stomach meridian (the energy pathway related to the energetic field of the stomach) runs up the front of the body and wraps around the eyes. If there is an imbalance in this "route" or pathway, a person may experience symptoms in their stomach but also their sinuses, because both areas share that energy flow. Another example is the gallbladder meridian, or pathway. While it governs and feeds the energy of the gallbladder, it also runs through the knees. It's not uncommon to have knee pain while experiencing an energy blockage in the gallbladder.

Disease and illness may manifest as chemical or physical imbalances, but they originate as "kinks" in the energy system. In fact, imbalances in the subtle energy field can be detected before symptoms arise in the physical body. All the organs, cells, and tissues in the body have an energetic frequency. Our thoughts have a frequency. Your body's energy system works in patterns that can be manipulated and changed. This means that by understanding and practicing with just a few principles, you'll see how you can access, improve, and eventually optimize these energies for your healing.

While various factors such as food and pollution have been shown to affect the vibrational frequency of the body, my own research led me to the work of Bruce Lipton, PhD. Dr. Lipton is a cellular biologist and author of the *New York Times* bestseller *The Biology of Belief: Unleashing the Power of Consciousness, Matter, and Miracles.* He is a leader in the field of epigenetics, the study of how our biology, including genetic factors, adapt to our environment. His work is based largely on the effects of stress on the human body, and their link to disease and illness. Dr. Lipton shares a critical message through his work: the body's physiology has the ability to respond and adapt to thoughts and emotions. You are not controlled by your genetic makeup. Instead, which genes are turned "on" and which are turned "off" is a process largely determined by your thoughts, emotions, and perceptions.

This offers incredible hope to all of us because it means we have more power than we ever may have believed to affect our lives. It is clear now that we are not hostages of our genes, bad luck, bad experiences, or fate. Our well-being is linked to our attitudes and perceptions.

These types of findings brought me to the conclusion that stress could be the single most influential factor of many disease processes and psychological challenges we face. In an effort to heal fully, I had tried every detox, diet, and medical treatment, and I eventually realized there was nothing left to correct except myself. Since wildly chasing bacteria, viruses, mold, parasites, and my own unruly cells didn't seem to be effective, I integrated what I learned from Dr. Lipton and focused instead on my energetic and emotional health. I knew of many people who had been bitten by ticks or exposed to similar things, yet they were not experiencing the same deep level of illness. I knew deep down, in spite of all other factors, that if I could get my mind, body, and spirit strong enough, it would be my best defense against all else.

## The Stress Mess

Stress is something I used to think of as running around trying to get my to-do list done, working hard, and dealing with the ups and downs of life. But I learned how very inaccurate that perspective is. The types of stress that create the most impact on our bodies does not come from rushing to get to work, having too much laundry, and more. It comes from physiological stress. Physiological stress comes from the body being in a heightened state of panic or fear, often called the fight, flight, or freeze pattern.

Sometimes, new clients come to me and say they are experiencing panic attacks, illness, or other challenges from doing "too much," working too hard, and running on empty for too long. And while this pattern of pushing ourselves past our limits is certainly an energy drain, the "doing" isn't the real problem. The *reason* we are pushing is the problem. Forcing ourselves to move at a pace that clashes with our spirit, or who we really are, is the core issue. The reasons we are living this way are where the true work lies.

I'll use myself as an example to demonstrate this point. I love to do, do, do. Part of it is my personality and that's just fine. I love to have a few projects going, read two books at once, and sometimes become completely lost in something. But this aspect of my personality is not what created unease and illness in my body. The *reasons* that I pushed myself too hard did. Back in the day, I often pushed because I wanted to be successful, perfect, and in control of everything in my life. These reasons are what catapulted me into the fight, flight, or freeze response. These reasons caused illness.

Humans are pretty darn resilient creatures. We can do a whole lot before we break. But we cannot clash against our spirit or the true nature of who we are. We just don't get away with that for too long.

Stress, or the fight, flight, or freeze response, is governed by a specific energy force in the body called the *triple warmer* meridian. I like to think of the triple warmer meridian as an inner protective "papa bear." When we hold unresolved emotional experiences in our bodies, we can become suspended in a place where the triple warmer meridian is in a state of panic or overdrive. It is not the stress itself that is necessarily a danger, but our bodies' reactions to that stress. In this fight, flight, or freeze state, the triple warmer meridian is doing everything it can to protect us (like a papa bear does for his cub), but it drains energy from the spleen, which supports the immune system. The triple warmer meridian also governs habits. When the triple warmer meridian is on high alert, it resists change in an effort to keep us safe. This is one reason that when we are in a state of stress, it can be so darn difficult to change habits. We often find ourselves resisting help, rebelling against things we know would be good for us, and abandoning self-care. It is because our triple warmer meridian's resistance to change is working as a form of self-sabotage, perceiving anything new or different as more stress.

When this energy dynamic is at play, the following physiological stress reactions are also taking place:

- Blood is shunted away from the gastrointestinal tract, spleen, and other non-vital organs.
- The body makes additional glucose.
- The immune system becomes suppressed, in part through the production of high cortisol levels brought on by the release of adrenaline.
- The areas of the brain related to short- and long-term memory are affected.
- Heart rate and blood pressure increase.

Stress hormones have been found to inhibit the production of anti-inflammatory cytokines and increase the production of pro-inflammatory cytokines. Cytokines are specific proteins that are responsible for signaling between cells to trigger the inflammation process in response to danger and decrease the process when the stress is over.

While stress is usually seen as a negative, it's important to point out that stress can be beneficial if we need the surge of chemicals to help us fight (defend ourselves), flight (escape the situation), or freeze (blend in or hide) to avoid danger. A great example of how the stress response should work is what happens in the wild. Animals exhibit this behavior (tigers "fight," rabbits "freeze," and antelope take "flight") but then shake, tremble, or otherwise let go of that state so they can continue in their environment. This pattern actually helps them stay alive. However, many of us get caught in this perpetual state, never releasing it from our system and returning to neutral.

A big challenge is that our systems cannot determine the difference between stresses due to an actual threat and those stemming from unresolved emotional conflict, unprocessed trauma (experiences), or an unhealthy emotional pattern like using negative self-talk.

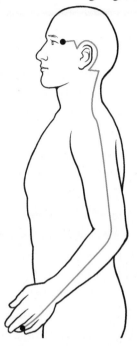

**Triple Warmer Meridian**

If we do not resolve these types of emotional patterns, our bodies may react in a harmful way. In my experience, physiological stress can be caused by anything that keeps us from relaxing or feeling safe in this world, emotionally or physically. This absolutely includes, above all else, not feeling safe to be our true selves. These are things we might not even realize are affecting us, and probably definitely not to the extent they are. In fact, it is completely possible to *be* stressed at a deep level but not feel stressed, as you would normally identify with it.

There are endless studies that cite stress as the dominating factor in many psychological conditions and physical diseases. However, stress itself isn't even so much the problem. It is how we *react* to those stressful influences that causes the internal stress, which closes us off to our well-being. In other words, the problem is our *relationship* with stress.

## The Question of "Why Me?"

When I first discovered all of this information you are now learning, I blamed myself. I questioned how some people, who had survived unspeakable traumas like war, could live happily and healthily into their nineties. And how someone like myself, who grew up with copious amounts of love and nothing I'd consider as traumatic as something like war, could end up where I was. Eventually, I realized that these struggles of mine were in no way due to flaws or failures of those who raised me, or something inherently wrong with me, either. They just *were*. Perhaps I was just born a sensitive soul. Perhaps this was simply meant to be my journey for a time. Without knowing the intricacies or answers, I let it all be okay. It was just time to move onward.

Now, I often get "why me?" from clients. *Why can't I handle things when I know others who have been through worse? Why can't I get over it already? What's wrong with me?* I want to explain this a bit further because it's so important.

First, there are emotional forces—beliefs, past experiences, perceptions, discomfort with who we are, and more—in each of us. These beliefs react with our energy system and this determines how we react to outside influences. Most of us have tried to change our external lives, but alas, we remain imbalanced, unhappy, or unhealthy. And while it's essential to listen to your heart in terms of leaving toxic relationships and making other changes that are good for your soul, it can be a faulty plan to rely on that completely. When you look at the effort and energy it takes to constantly try to control or adapt to situations around you—whether it be chasing viruses or trying to change stressful circumstances in life—you will find that this, in and of itself, is stressful. And you will learn that it is far easier to make any necessary changes that your soul desires when you feel better about yourself.

Second, there are two types of energies with which you may have come to this world. These are past-life energies and generational energies. Let me briefly explain.

## Past-Life Energies

The concept of past lives is built on the idea or belief that before you came here, to this earth, you lived many lives before. You had experiences, connections, and relationships that you still carry with you from those past lives that may be negatively affecting your experience here in this life. For example, perhaps in a past life you were a mother who lost her child in a car accident. It is possible that in this lifetime you will still hold some of the fears or memories in your energy field, which are impeding your experience now. This was not something I explored during my healing process, but it is something I have seen to be beneficial for clients to work on. While there are many professionals who specialize in past-life regression (a process of leading you back into that past life in order to heal it), I will teach you how I clear energies that come from past-life experiences.

## Generational Energies

Generational energies are energies you inherited from your ancestors. You might have heard various names for these energies, including *inherited energies* or *ancestral energies*. In the same way we can inherit genes or personality traits from our parents and ancestors, we sometimes inherit their energies, too. These energies can be in the form of unresolved emotion from experiences from their lives, beliefs, or fears. Many people who are carrying around heavy generational energies may feel like they've always had a cloud over their head. They may have a difficult time determining when it started or where it's from. They may describe it as not feeling like their own—and this is accurate because their body doesn't sense a point of origin for it. I see this often in families with heavy energy lineages, like Holocaust survivors. If you suspect this is relevant to you (and even if you don't), it's wise to explore it.

When you work with generational energies, it's important to know that everyone has them. There is no reason to be angry with your parents or ancestors. We can pass along lots of stuff to our kids and no one is immune. It's part of life to work this stuff out. While these energies may not be "ours," they are our responsibility to clear for ourselves. I believe that these energies keep getting passed down until they perhaps reach a person who is evolved and conscious enough to be capable of clearing them. This is a great opportunity for you to turn around a long-held familial pattern.

While past-life and generational energies can be important, it's essential that we don't get into a place of focusing primarily on them. I have never seen these energies be more important in the healing process than one's own experiences, beliefs, and other patterns. They are certainly worth exploring, but do not allow yourself to use them as a distraction from your own "stuff."

Perhaps it's your own life experience that has brought you to this place, or perhaps you have some of the "born with" energies and they are affecting you. It's likely a mix of both. If you are not healing or finding happiness like you thought you would, or like you thought you should, it doesn't mean you're broken. In fact, it means you are exceptional. You are breaking through, breaking free, breaking open in ways that could happen only by having your patience and persistence challenged. Vitamin B or detoxing or the strongest treatment on earth could not do for you what this process is doing for you.

But the real answer to the "why me?" question is that the answer doesn't matter. You are where you are for some reason that you might not fully understand. But this I'm sure of: the universe, and your body, will not let you do what you've been doing any longer—living small or whatever else you've been up to. This is both the human burden and the gift. This is meant to be your path. Not forever, though. You get to move on from here.

## Change Your Relationship with Stress

The body has the incredible ability both to protect and defend itself (via the fight, flight, or freeze response) and to heal and repair itself. The only catch is that these processes cannot happen simultaneously. The body can only settle into full healing mode once we take it out of its crisis mode, or sustained stress state. This does not in any way mean that you have to be stress-free to heal. It simply means that it is your work to do what you can to make your body feel safe enough to do so.

The best way to get the body to relax enough to heal is by turning off the fight, flight, or freeze pattern. In other words, we need to convince the triple warmer meridian that it's safe to come out of intense papa bear mode. A proven method of doing this is by turning on the *relaxation response*, a term coined by Dr. Herbert Benson, Associate Professor of Medicine at Harvard Medical School.[2] The relaxation response is a physical state of relaxation that can be achieved by participating in activities such as yoga, energy healing, acupuncture, prayer, meditation, qi gong, and many other modalities—all of which create the opposite effect of the fight, flight, or freeze response. In fact, the relaxation response is so powerful that you can see its potential in the common phenomenon where people who have food allergies will often see a dramatic decrease or disappearance in reactions while they are on vacation. This is because their body is not being triggered into a stress response in the same way it usually is at home. Perhaps they feel less fearful to be themselves in a place where nobody knows them, or their boss is not triggering the "I'm not good enough" feeling that causes stress, and more.

My own process, which you'll be practicing throughout this entire book, is effective because we are always working directly with releasing that root emotional imbalance and its relationship to stress in the energy system. Utilizing an approach called *energy psychology*, which is the basis of this book, does this. Energy psychology simply refers to techniques that specifically address the relationship between our energy system and our emotions, thoughts, and behavior. Accessing and working with our energy system in this way gives us the opportunity to change our relationship to stress, which helps us become the most integrated, joyful version of ourselves.

Energy work gives us a tool to talk our triple warmer meridian (aka the papa bear meridian) off the ledge and onto more stable ground. It

---

2. Herbert Benson, MD, *RelaxationResponse.org*, www.relaxationresponse.org.

is only then that the body can move from a place of defense and protection to the place of instigating its powerful self-healing ability.

In order to heal fully and completely, we need to change our physiological response to stress. When you do this, you will not be a prisoner of worry, fearing that stress can take you down. I remember doctors telling me, even as I healed, that I would always be at high risk for relapse if I got stressed. If I caught a cold or the flu, did too much, or ate sugar, I would end up sick again, they'd say. This is a very common experience for many, and I was informed of it in only well-meaning ways; however, this became not only a personal belief of mine but also a stress in and of itself because I ended up feeling out of control and helpless. *I can't handle stress. I'll get sick again if I catch a cold. Relapse is inevitable.*

It tortured me, but it didn't have to, because I eventually learned that once you do the inner work and strengthen your being at a core level, which includes changing your relationship with stress, you are no longer the fragile person you might have been before. It's essential to update your mental records about this. You can take a little roughing around. You can get well, and stay well, even when you have too much to do, eat some sugar, or catch a cold.

To be completely empowered (and successful!), it is far more intelligent to shift our relationships and reactions to external influences, so we can remain stable even on shaky ground.

## The Benefit of Self-Healing

Don't fear if you are sitting frozen wondering how you will ever get from where you are now to a place where you can express and live from your true self while feeling calm and balanced.

It's likely to happen in comfortable baby steps instead of giant leaps. As you'll be learning more about shortly, feeling out of control is one of the biggest triggers for us feeling unsafe in this world. Self-healing immediately works on counteracting that deep-seated feeling with every application you practice. In essence, it reverses helplessness. By embracing self-healing, you will learn to feel safe in your own hands, affirming the message of "I can be okay," no matter what, and "I can help myself!"

In other words, the sheer act of taking your healing into your own hands sends a strong message to the body of safety and capability, actually reversing the fight, flight, or freeze response. The practice of self-healing acts as its own healing modality. You will soon come to see that you are the key to a process of which you felt so wildly out of control.

The only requirement for success is that we need to do our own work. Even while using the support of medicine or other alternatives, we cannot excuse ourselves from the biggest part of the process. People often feel pressure to choose one way or another—Western medicine or natural healing. But the truth is that there is no right or wrong path. We just have to meet our chosen medicine halfway. Even for those who prefer to use natural healing, medical intervention does not have to feel like failure in any way. Treatment often gives us time to heal the real wounds. Any healing approach can be beneficial for us when we find a way to feel good about it. The bottom line is that we need to become an environment where healing happens. We need to clean up our soil. And the best way I know to do that is by addressing your whole self—mind (mental patterns), body (physical self, including energetic patterns in the body), *and* spirit (the energy of who you really are at the core).

## An Introduction to My Three-Part Approach to Healing

You may remember the tree analogy from earlier. Deep and permanent healing comes from cleaning up the soil of your life so that you can be who you really are. Everything that will help you heal ultimately comes down to that one focus, and that's what my work is based on. Here, I'm going to briefly outline my approach to healing that we'll be going through together in section II.

### Part One: Surrender, Accept, and Flow

Before you can even begin to heal, you have to surrender to where you are as your starting point. You have to be able to look at yourself as that tree with some brittle leaves and soil that could use love, and become okay with where you currently are. Being right where you are and being at peace with that is a required part of the healing process. Actually, it's a required part of life. I know it sucks and you're trying desperately to get to a better place, but learning to accept exactly where you are now in all of your ungraceful glory is super-duper important. Learning to forgive yourself, laugh at yourself, and stop beating yourself up about every little thing is, ironically, part of why you're here. You *must* learn to be easier on yourself. You must stop wasting your energy fighting so darn hard. Fixing things might be your goal, but learning to feel better about the things you want to fix is an essential part of your journey.

Learning the art of surrender is essential, because in that space, there is great opportunity to create a foundation for your healing. This includes starting to work with energy and thought patterns. Through this, you can practice being gentle with yourself. You will need this skill, because a being who is berated will not easily heal. You know how it feels when other people have done this to you? All the years of trying to unravel the messages you got from parents, teachers, and others? "You should do more." "You should be more." "Hurry up and succeed." Well, you need to start doing the opposite of that. You need to learn to be lighter on yourself. It's a requirement for well-being. Instead, say things like, "It's okay, I have time." "I can relax." "I'm doing just fine." I promise, it will make a magical difference in your life.

### Part Two: Identify Blockages

There are several things that block our healing process. In order to heal, each and every part of our being must be aligned with being well. While this seems obvious, the majority of my clients have some big resistance to being well. In other words, often at a subconscious level that they're not aware of, they aren't in full alignment with their own healing. Being in alignment means *wanting* to heal, feeling *deserving* of healing, knowing you are *able* to heal, being *ready* to heal, and more. If at any level, either consciously or unconsciously, part of you is resistant to overcoming your challenge, it's going to be like climbing Mount Rainier against the wind. Maybe it already has been this difficult, and now you know why.

Let me show you this concept in action. Let's say you started experiencing panic attacks right before the school spelling bee in eighth grade, an event at which you were convinced you'd fail. And because of that panic attack, your teacher let you sit out and just watch your classmates instead of participating. Can you see how now, even many years later, a part of you may not want to overcome these panic attacks because you learned that they protect you? Perhaps part of you, even if just subconsciously, still feels that you need the panic attacks to help you get out of scary things—like being humiliated or embarrassed by your peers. This type of scenario could prevent you from being in alignment with full healing. Alignment with our goal is something that we all need to pay very close attention to. Blocks that cause resistance to healing show up most commonly in people who experience "nothing working," or every treatment making them feel worse.

The body's language is also a great indicator of what emotional energy from the past or what current patterns need to be addressed and cleared for full and complete healing. The body's symptoms are full of clues, messages, and metaphors that can help us identify exactly what needs to be healed inside. A huge key to healing, as you'll learn, is actually finding what is standing in your way of it. Once you do that, you'll be well on your way.

### Part Three: Change Your Relationship with Stress
Stress is a buzzword we all hear often. But remember, stress itself is not actually the gigantic problem that we think it is. It's your relationship with stress that is the problem. It's important to identify and transform your relationship with stress instead of trying to eliminate stress itself. If you are experiencing physical symptoms, we can safely assume that your immune system is being suppressed—and your relationship with stress is a big reason why. And, if you are experiencing only emotional challenges, well, that makes it even more apparent that this stress factor is important to address.

The stressful reactions in your body come from things like these:

- Unprocessed experiences
- Harmful beliefs

- Unhealthy emotional patterns
- Fear

All of these aspects affect how you relate and respond in your life. Changing your relationship with stress by working with these main areas will have a huge impact on your life. Huge.

Now that you have a rundown of the process, it's time to move on and get into some practice. Next, in section II, we'll be doing just that.

# A Tried-and-True
# Healing Process

\* \* \* \* \* \* \* \* \* \* \* \* \* \* \*

# Part One

# Surrender, Accept, and Flow

Imagine you are swimming in the ocean, a mile out. The sky is blue and the world feels beautiful. But a minute later, everything changes. *Where did these clouds come from?* you think. *Why is the water so rough?* You start to fear for your safety, and you start to fight. You kick and flail and use every ounce of energy to stay afloat. In the first five minutes you have exhausted yourself, and now your head is barely above water.

What would happen, though, if you changed your approach? What if you surrendered to and accepted your current reality? *I am in a scary ocean. These waves are big. I cannot swim against them at the moment. I am doing the best that I can. I want to fix this, but I can't right now.* What if you turned on your back, stared up at that big, angry sky, and just let go?

Do you know what would happen?

I do. You'd float. And then you'd flow more easily in any direction.

There is something that *always* happens when you surrender and accept exactly where you are, find a way to be okay with it (and yourself), and stop fighting. You release yourself from at least half the hard work you've been doing. You have the energy to be with yourself through it. You have the opportunity to soften up and relax. You give up the "fight," and because of it, you actually start to be free with far less effort than ever before.

In part one, we will be exploring the importance of surrendering to where you currently are, even if you aren't where you want to be. You will learn why it's essential, and techniques to help you actually do this. You'll be able to use this space you create to work gently with yourself, and to build a solid foundation for your healing. You cannot hate your way to anywhere, especially healing. You just can't. Once you give up the fighting energy, you will have a new and more grounded starting point for yourself. You will also discover how to take baby steps in directing your thinking *about* where you are, which will aid you in making things feel so much more comfortable until you can reach where you really want to be.

\* \* \* \* \* \* \* \* \* \* \* \* \* \*

### Chapter Three

# It's Time to Stop Fighting

*It's healthy to say uncle when your bone's about to break.*
—JONATHAN FRANZEN, *HOW TO BE ALONE*

Surrender is a word we interpret to mean giving up. Surrendering to where you are now, though, is very different from giving up. It's the opposite. It's acknowledging the starting point of "here." In this chapter, you'll understand what surrender really entails, read examples of what it means to surrender, and learn important techniques to help you surrender. By using the techniques of Chanting and of Graceful Begging (my version of non-denominational prayer), you'll be well on your way to not just understanding surrender but actually doing it, too.

While it's a very human reaction, when facing challenges, to immediately find a way to escape them or hurry through them, there is immense importance in being in the place you most want to run from. Surrender does not mean giving up; it's simply releasing the energy of struggle and deciding to heal instead of fight. Being where you are is incredibly vital because it, too, is part of your healing. You are not here, in this place, to find that perfect doctor who will reconstruct your body and extract all of the bad feelings you have. You are here to talk to your soul. You are here to practice being kind to yourself, no matter where you are. You are here to transform your life into the enjoyable experience it is meant to be.

Surrendering is the act of simply allowing what *is* to be okay for now. Getting to a place of not feeling so bad about feeling bad is a massive first step. When we surrender to just "being," we immediately put ourselves in a state of ease. When we are at ease, we are in healing mode. We can get stuck in the mindset that healing is "doing," when often it's a matter of "being" instead. Rigid action is not always necessary or beneficial. Healing can find its way into your experience through something inspiring you read, a gentle awareness, finding compassion for yourself, or a silent moment that brings new insight or guidance. These types of healing experiences are impossible to have if we are in mental or physical overdrive.

Through the process of surrendering to the discomfort that life brings, we are also able to honor the incredible opportunity that I call "the silver lining of suffering." We get to release all that no longer serves us and transform ourselves into all we are meant to be. We get to come out of this stronger and better in ways we wouldn't have ever dreamt for ourselves. Jenny Rush of the Lyme Thriving website said something that I couldn't say any better: "Illness and suffering seem to go hand in hand. However, if we turn to face our suffering thoughts, dig down through them to their source, they dissipate as we come into a fresh clearing where our essence abides. Illness and the struggle with it can be used to find our way in and out. The illness is already there, might as well use it rather than be used by it. You deserve to know the wonder of who you are."

But to use this journey, you must surrender to it fully, just for the moment.

## Examples of Surrender Experiences

The energy of surrender itself has proved, in my own journey, to be exceptionally healing. When I was first diagnosed with Lyme disease, there was a very concentrated effort by my doctors to "fight and kill" the bacteria. From the day the tests came back, it was all about the eradication of the "invader." I'm not sure if it was by example or of my own doing, but soon I found myself, too, in "killer" mode. My doctors and I would pow-wow about "obliterating" the disease, "beating" it, and "kicking" it to the curb. I sought out the strongest medications and the most powerful treatments, and embraced the extreme struggle of each protocol because I perceived that the harshness of it all kept me "winning." I learned everything under the sun about how to kill the various viruses and bacteria in my body, and I used my life as a control center to do so. I had charts and supplements and drugs, and controlled each and every move I made to use my weapons in the war on Lyme. In part, this is the Western medicine mentality, but I also adopted it because I had no other awareness of how things could be.

In India, I had an experience that provided the backdrop for my love affair with surrender. I wouldn't fully understand and embrace it until later, but I now see that the seeds were planted during this time.

Each day in the hospital, I panicked during IV time. The protocol and practices varied greatly in comparison to standard practices in the US. My fears heightened because I was so used to dictating every little part of my medical care at home, from self-injecting my prescription antibiotics to suggesting what blood tests my doctors should order. Every time it was time for an IV in this new country, my body would tighten and I would obsessively watch every move the nurses made, compare things to home, and create abundant scenarios in my head of things that could go wrong during the process.

Then, one random day, in a moment of deliberate surrender, I chose to just give up. I turned my head away and ... I let the fuck go. I decided that if I were to die because someone was putting in an IV that wasn't "my way," so be it! I just couldn't keep it up anymore; the struggle to fight "what was" was draining my last ounce of energy. In fact, this was a pattern of mine that my body had been trying to warn me about for a long time. But it wasn't until then, suddenly and seemingly out of nowhere, that I really got what my fight was doing to me. It was making my life hard—and healing even harder.

Every day from then on, I got to practice surrendering when it was IV time. *Deep breath, turn head.* This ritual went on for weeks before I started to settle into the routine, slowly coming to terms with the fact that I probably wasn't going to die from either the IV or the letting go. It was quite possibly my first baby step in the direction of freedom. I saw in that moment that I had the ability to create relief for myself, just by choosing to relax. Later, I'd come back to this example many times as a reminder of the energy I could save by surrendering again and again, even and especially when it was uncomfortable.

Now I realize that all the years I was eagerly fueling "the war on Lyme"—symptom tracking, trying to control each moment, and angrily "beating" the disease—I was actually throwing the energy of a fight into my very own body. I was stuck in a process of fighting against everything, including *myself*. There is no way, when you hold the energy of attack and fight, not to absorb that into all of your cells, the diseased ones and the healthy ones too.

The act of surrender will take great courage. You are going to have to do this very difficult thing, and that is, let go of *how you thought things should be*—just for now. That won't be easy, either. But to set the wheels in motion, you need only ask yourself this one question, as many times as it takes: *Do I want to fight my way to healing or do I want to flow there?* It's all in your energy. Choose wisely.

I'd like to share one of my favorite client examples of surrender as inspiration for you.

When I first started working with Susan, she was more frustrated than any client I had ever seen. She had a list that was pages and pages long of every doctor, symptom, ailment, medication, treatment, and approach that had filled the last ten years of her life. She didn't understand why she wasn't better; neither did anyone she'd gone to for help. The fight that was in this woman was fierce, and for good reason. But the problem was, she was so sick of being sick that she was wearing herself out trying not to be sick. She hated herself every day that she wasn't healed, which put her into fight, flight, or freeze mode—and then made it even harder for her to heal. We spent several sessions just working with some techniques (which you will learn shortly) to get her to a place of feeling okay with where she was and being nice to herself in spite of not being well. While she wasn't sure about it at first, she woke up one day and said she just felt different. When I asked her to explain it, she said she felt clear and calm for the first time in ten years.

It was like she had been relieved of this enormous pressure-filled job to "hurry up and get somewhere else or be someone else."

This was the beginning of Susan's path toward feeling better not only emotionally but physically, too. It certainly wasn't coincidental that once she started to accept herself and her starting point, she freed up energy for her healing.

Sometimes when we don't like how our lives are looking, we get to decide to take things for what and how they are, right now. And often that's exactly what we need.

Knowing it's beneficial to surrender and knowing how to surrender are vastly different things, so let me offer you some ideas on just how to do it. The end game here is to become comfortable enough with where you are that your body can relax. That's it. Simple!

### Chanting

My first introduction to chanting was in Delhi, where you can hear its reverberation throughout the city. Kneeling in front of something shrine-like, with my sister-in-law Tatiana, who was visiting from the States, we were strangers to it. There was no opportunity to ask questions or express our emotions before the chanting service began.

The energy shifted around me as we began to follow along, first slowly and then much faster. *Nam Myoho Renge Kyo*. This, I learned, was the practice of *daimoku*—chanting with specific words that reveal one's state of inner Buddhahood.

Our synchronous chanting created a steady hum in the room. The presence of something transformational was palpable. When I finally opened my eyes after losing complete awareness of time, I suddenly felt at peace with where I was in my journey.

We were told to continue the practice and stay "aware of miracles." We packed up to leave, still buzzing with energy. Still unsure of the significance of the experience on the way home, Tatiana and I agreed it was, at a minimum, super cool. When I got back to my hospital room, I googled "daimoku" and found that we'd just chanted words from Tina Turner's religion. I watched a clip of her from *Larry King Live*, and her seamless chanting became my new aspiration.

I chanted whenever I was terrified or angry or simply lost. In times of pain, the chants welled up from within me. Chanting helped me surrender because it both distracted me from the fight and kept me present, actually making the moments bearable.

For thousands of years, singing or chanting has been a spiritual practice among many cultures and religions. With each word, chanting creates special vibratory sounds that hold the power to clear energy. The repetition directs the mind out of its usual craziness and into a higher vibration. That vibration rings throughout the body, clearing blocks. This is important because fighting against and having resistance to where you are can be caused by an energy imbalance and can also create one.

Because every molecule, cell, tissue, organ, gland, bone, and so on in our bodies has its own specific vibration, any sound or vibration that interplays with those can have a profound impact on us. Because we often feel uncomfortable if we can't "do" something to change our situation immediately, the added benefit of chanting is that it gives us something to "do" that is healthy. It offers us active practice to help us shift away from trying so darn hard to fix things right now.

The repetition of a phrase is called a *mantra*. In many practices, a mantra is chosen based on the name of God, but you can use any positive phrase, from ancient religious or spiritual words to affirmations that you are in alignment with. Words are just energy, like everything else. Because of that, they have a direct impact on our bodies. With this knowledge in mind, it would be beneficial for you to choose a phrase for your chanting that either feels good to you or means something to you that helps you feel good.

Because there are endless possibilities for mantras, my list is wildly incomplete but is still a great starting place. You'll find your own chanting groove in no time.

**Om**—Om is a word that comes from the Sanskrit language and is often described as the sound of the universe or the sound of creation. You can think of it as a symbolic "seed" from which anything can come. While it has roots in Hinduism and Buddhism, it's a word that can be chanted by those from all faiths.

**Om Mani Padme Hum**—This is a Tibetan mantra and it means, roughly, "Hail to the jewel in the lotus." The jewel in this case is the Buddha of Compassion, and self-directed compassion is always beneficial for our healing.

**Ho'oponopono**—This Hawaiian mantra means "I love you, I'm sorry, Please forgive me, Thank you." These are all wonderful things to say to yourself!

**Nam Myoho Renge Kyo**—While this mantra translates as "I devote myself to the Lotus Sutra," Nichiren, its creator, encouraged the chanting of *Nam Myoho Renge Kyo* as a practice by which chanters could spark their inherent Buddha nature—strengthening their capacity for wisdom, courage, confidence, vitality, and compassion. This is the first one I learned, and I just love the feel of it.

**Om Gum Ganapataye Namaha**—This is a salutation to the Hindu Lord Ganesha (the elephant god), said to be the "remover of obstacles." The meaning behind this one is soothing. Who doesn't want some of their obstacles removed, right?

**I am**—While this phrase is powerful on its own—because as I interpret it, it means "I am enough"—you can easily add an affirmation to this, making it *I am getting stronger, I am peace, I am healing*, and more.

**I can**—*I can* is a very impactful mantra, as it allows us to remind ourselves of our infinite power and capability. Some of my favorite extensions for this one are *I can handle this* and *I can heal*.

**All is well**—This is a favorite I learned from studying the works of Louise Hay. Even during the times I didn't believe it, I sensed it was true.

**Be here now**—This one keeps us in the present moment, where it is impossible to regret, resent, or worry, as can tend to happen when we focus on the past or the future.

**This too shall pass**—This mantra is a personal favorite. I remind myself often that everything is fleeting, from this time in my life to this emotion and beyond. Everything blows just like the wind and moves, if I allow it.

**I am well, I am whole**—Taken from the little book *Scientific Healing Affirmations* by Paramahansa Yogananda, author of the famous *Autobiography of a Yogi*, this affirmation has become one of my all-time favorites. When we are experiencing illness or challenge, we tend to see ourselves as broken. This affirmation reverses that trained thinking.

**Thank you**—Gratitude is one of the highest healing vibrations. You may hear of stories where gratitude alone has helped people heal from incredible challenges. Many of us have a hard time being grateful when we are in the midst of struggle. However, saying these simple words over and over is powerful in itself. If English is not your primary language, I suggest you say it in whatever language has the most meaning to you.

**Bird by bird**—Author Anne Lamott tells a powerful story in her book *Bird By Bird: Some Instructions on Writing and Life*. Her brother, who was ten years old, was struggling to finish a report on birds for school by the next day. Her father sat down with him, put his arm around her brother's shoulder, and said, 'Bird by bird, buddy. Just take it bird by bird.' The bird-by-bird concept is extremely comforting. You can chant it to release the overwhelming feeling of needing to fix everything, especially all at once.

Before you begin chanting to help you feel better about where you are at this moment, I suggest you set an intention. Here is my short-and-sweet intention prayer for surrender chanting:

*Universe and inner being, please allow these vibrations to move through me, clearing away resistance to where I am in this moment.*
*Help me find peace.*
*And so it is done.*

You will begin and remain chanting (repeating the phrase in whatever rhythm feels good to you) for as long as you can. When first learning a chant that's not in English, it's sometimes helpful to look them up online and listen to a video or an audio so you can hear how they are chanted. You can also chant right along. It's okay to start slowly. When I first started, I was a very short-term chanter. I lasted only a minute or two before I became bored or distracted. But I grew from there. I now set my phone timer for several minutes at a time and then continue from there, resetting it again and again.

Chants often start softly and slowly, then get louder and faster. However, chant so the vibration feels good to your body because that will be the most healing. Always chant quietly if you are lying down or if you are very low on energy. If you find it difficult to sit down and chant, you can also do it while pacing or walking.

Chanting is so easy that it almost feels too simple. Whatever approach you decide to try, remember to find your own rhythm and go your own way.

> *Tip:* I love to use chanting for surrender. However, chanting while focusing on moving energy blockages in specific parts of the body is excellent, too. Remember how the vibration of your chant moves through your cells? You can really use that to your advantage by directing your focus to whatever in your body or mind needs it most. Simply set your intention or say a short prayer stating what you intend for the chanting vibration to clear. Choose a mantra that feels good to you, and chant away!

## Graceful Begging

While I didn't grow up praying, and even rebelled against the idea, sometimes during my deepest, darkest days, I just begged. I called out in the dark and I begged for help from no one in particular. Over and over when I reached places of despair, I'd beg. Not gracefully (at the time), but from a place of total rawness, with a mixture of tears and snot dripping down my face. When I had sunken into places I believed I couldn't pull myself from, I'd reach for this and it would bring me the reprieve I so desperately needed.

Just knowing that this was available to me, void of rules and full of organic and creative liberty, helped to solidify my love affair with it. Over time, it became a dedicated practice where I could feel my energy shift even before I started. I began to wonder why. *How did this help?*

It's all in the surrendering. It's the throwing of it from your hands and your heart and soul and simply moving beyond that heaviness of "I have to fix this in this moment." It's the energy of handing it over to a force greater than yourself.

In the practice of surrendering, we are eliciting the ever-so-important relaxation response. Surrender is the ultimate space for relaxation, for there is nothing to do but simply be. In fact, I believe that the positive benefits linked to prayer, which are now being studied more than ever, are based largely upon the relaxation response, too.

My original practice of screaming out and crying is now the technique of *Graceful Begging*, which has a resemblance to prayer but is free from any negative religious associations. In fact, at some point I discovered that the word *prayer* comes from the Latin *precarius*, which means "obtained by begging." It makes this practice available to and relatable for everyone. It works best for me when I'm in a place of total willingness to let go—which often isn't until I've exhausted all of my options for trying to control my current circumstance.

While the goal of this practice, whether praying or begging, is not necessarily to induce healing, it seems to be a common byproduct.

The Gerontological Society of America published a study of the role of prayer in psychological recovery following surgery. The effects of private prayer on a group of 151 older patients following cardiac surgery were observed.[3] Results showed that most patients pray about their post-operative problems and that prayer seems to significantly decrease depression and general distress.

---

3. Amy L. Ai, PhD, Ruth E. Dunkle, PhD, Christopher Peterson, PhD, and Steven F. Bolling, MD, "The Role of Private Prayer in Psychological Recovery Among Midlife and Aged Patients Following Cardiac Surgery," *The Gerontologist* Vol. 38,
No. 5 (Oct. 1998): 591–601, http://gerontologist.oxfordjournals.org/content/38/5/591.full.pdf.

A study funded by the National Institutes of Health showed that people who prayed at least once a day were 40 percent less likely to have high blood pressure than those who did so infrequently.[4]

A study conducted by researchers at the University of Cincinnati revealed that inner-city kids with asthma who prayed and meditated had fewer symptoms than those who did not.[5]

As I healed, I turned much of the begging I did into more formulated, purposeful requests that I made and then let go of. Here, I'm offering you some of my own scripts that have a little more method than my original scream-it-out-to-no-one madness.

Let this practice be a way for you to ask for help from outside of your current control, for surrendering, allowing you to feel better about where you actually are. It will make it far easier to then flow or float into the next space you are meant to be in.

Just remember to be gentle with yourself during this process. You have been conditioned by society, the media, and probably the medical community to "fight." We have the "war" on cancer, we "beat" heart disease, and the list goes on. We are subconsciously being trained to fight till the death—our own death, if necessary. Changing takes bravery. We are all born brave, though. You'll do just great.

Most importantly, feel free to beg loud and proud and repeat the words that feel best to your soul. Place your hands over your heart, a calming position for most, then take a big, deep breath and recite any or all of the following suggestions. Take deep breaths in between each round, and repeat until you feel relief.

**Directed at the universe:**

*Dear universe, please help me surrender to where I am in this moment. Please help me surrender to this process. Please help me trust that I am*

4. Harold G. Koenig, MD, "Religion and Medicine II: Religion, Mental Health, and Related Behaviors," *The International Journal of Psychiatry in Medicine* Vol. 31, No. 1 (2001): 97–109, www.rish.ch/mm/Koenig_%282001%29_Rel _and_Medi_II_Rel_Mental_Health_and_Related_Behaviours_IJPM_31% 281%29.pdf.

5. Richard Schiffman, "Why People Who Pray Are Healthier Than Those Who Don't," *Huffington Post*, January 18, 2012, www.huffingtonpost.com/richard -schiffman/why-people-who-pray-are-heathier_b_1197313.html.

*exactly where I need to be, and when I need to be somewhere else, I will be guided in getting there. I leave it all with you. Thank you and so it is done!*

### Directed at your own inner being or higher power:

*Dear inner being, please help to reassure me that I am okay exactly where I am at this moment. Please help me release this energy of overwhelm. I need to do nothing more than allow what "should be" to unfold for me. Thank you and so it is done!*

### A "graceful begging" with no particular receiver in mind:

*In this moment, I ask to release all resistance to where I am. I ask to release myself of all fighting energy so that I can harness it for my healing. I ask to feel that I am okay right where I am at this moment, and trust that clarity, ease, and abundance are making their way to me. Thank you and so it is done!*

Now that you've got the hang of it, feel free to come up with your own versions of graceful begging. Alternatively, if my original ape-style craziness feels like it would be a better energy release, then beg and cry and scream out loud. I can tell you from experience that definitely works, too. When the need arises, go for it!

\* \* \* \* \* \* \* \*

You now have two tools to help you start your surrender process: Chanting and Graceful Begging. In part three, you will learn Emotional Freedom Technique (EFT), which applies most fully to changing your relationship to stress. However, if you are still struggling with surrender, EFT tapping may be a handy technique for this as well. It may also be helpful to remember the story about my IV experience, because when all else fails, you really can choose to let go.

Now that you understand what good a healthy dose of surrender can be, let me reassure you of something. From this place of feeling more comfortable with where you currently are, you will see that it's easier to flow naturally to a better feeling place. In the next chapter, you will learn how, from this more relaxed state, to build a solid foundation for your healing.

*Chapter Four*

\* \* \* \* \* \* \* \* \* \* \* \* \* \*

# Create a Solid
# Healing Foundation

*The way I see it, there are just two things we need to know:*
*The universe has our back. Everything is going to turn out okay.*
—PAM GROUT, *E-SQUARED*

While you are in this place of learning to be okay with where you are, there is space for something wonderful to happen. In the absence of the constant-fighting energy, you will now be able to create a solid foundation for your healing work. In this chapter, we'll be setting the stage for all the shifts and changes to come. You'll learn four effective ways to create a foundation to build on. None of these things require giant leaps of time or energy. If you're willing to take baby steps, and take them consistently, you're already winning.

In this chapter, you'll gain tools to do the following:

1. Correct your body's polarities
2. Encourage a crossover energy pattern
3. Balance your thymus gland
4. Inch your way to better thoughts and feelings

Addressing these elements is like pouring a solid cement foundation before building a house. The more stable the foundation, the easier it is to make that house stand tall, right?

Let me show you how this works.

## 1: Correct Your Body's Polarities

Just like magnets, our bodies have both a north and a south pole, the south being the bottom of our feet and the north being the top of our head. In fact, every organ and cell in the body is polarized. Imagine each cell like a tiny little battery. Generally speaking, the top surfaces of your body (your stomach, tops of feet, tops of hands) should have a positive polarity and your body's bottom surfaces (your back, bottoms of your feet, palms of your hands) should have a negative polarity. However, they are often reversed or switched. In simple terms, it is like your batteries are in backward. When this happens, we don't function well and can be resistant to respond to energy work.

*Grounding* (sometimes called *earthing*) is essentially the practice of connecting yourself to both the earth's north and south poles. Grounding allows the natural healing properties and rhythms of the earth to correct the body's polarities.

Throughout history, humans have walked barefoot and slept on the ground. This process helped the body calibrate itself to the electrical rhythm of the earth, stabilizing the electrical current of organs, tissues, and cells. In other words, our batteries worked correctly. But our modern lifestyle—including the use of rubber and plastic-soled shoes and being almost constantly connected to electrical devices like cell phones and computers—has disconnected us from the earth's energy. Emerging research has now revealed a benefit to reconnecting with the vast supply of electrons on the surface of the earth. A study in the *Journal of Environmental and Public Health* concludes that reconnection with the earth's electrons has the potential to trigger positive physiological changes linked to stress.[6] The researchers discovered that grounding the human body can "strongly influence bioelectrical, bioenergetic, and biochemical processes that appear to have a significant modulating effect on chronic illnesses." In the study, changes in the subjects after grounding suggest a decrease in stress levels and a bal-

---

6. Gaétan Chevalier, et al., "Earthing: Health Implications of Reconnecting the Human Body to the Earth's Surface Electrons," *Journal of Environmental and Public Health* Vol. 2012 (Jan. 12, 2012), www.ncbi.nlm.nih.gov/pmc/articles /PMC3265077.

ancing of the autonomic nervous system (this system is the primary mechanism in control of the fight, flight, or freeze response).

Let me explain why this discovery is so essential to your healing foundation. Having reversed polarities, similarly to having batteries in backward, makes it hard for things to work correctly. This includes changing your belief system, retraining your thought patterns, and other positive changes you try to make. As an added benefit, remember that ever-so-important triple warmer meridian? The process of grounding also affects this energy dynamic. Grounding is a very gentle, natural way to coax the triple warmer meridian into relaxing. Our bodies already know how to use the earth's supply of electrons in order to balance. When the triple warmer meridian relaxes, you do, too. It is then far easier to change habits, stress patterns, and energy patterns than it would be in the state of fighting everything.

Grounding both the north and the south poles of the energy field completes an important electrical circuit in the body to help it function. I'm going to share two ways of doing this: outdoors and indoors.

### Grounding Outdoors

In order to ground both the north and the south poles of your body to the north and south poles of the earth, you can use the very simple technique of sitting against a tree. Find a tree, align your spine against it, and place your bare feet on the earth—either in dirt, sand (yes, I just gave you a prescription for the beach!), or grass. Hang out. That's it. The roots of the tree carry the body's energy down into the earth and then return it back up into the body. This is very effective for helping you complete a healthy energy circuit in your body. Fifteen to thirty minutes a day is ideal. Often, though, if I only have two or five minutes, I notice feeling better from that too.

If you don't have a tree to sit against, walking in grass (wet grass is even better) is a very powerful grounding technique as well.

> *Tip:* If you can't get your feet on something natural, unsealed concrete is a good grounding source. Concrete pools, because they are underground, are excellent as well.

## *Grounding Indoors*

For this exercise, you will need a stainless steel spoon. If you are unsure if it's stainless steel, you can check by looking for an imprint of "ss" on it.

The areas in between the tendons on the tops of the feet are places where lots of energy get stuck. Because of this, the feet can make it difficult to "draw up" a ground, which we need for healthy polarities. Using a stainless steel spoon, you can change that. Stainless steel possesses a mineral that aids in the break-up of congested energy. Using the rounded edge of the spoon on the tops of the feet, gently make big crisscross patterns with it. This will help break up energy in the tops of the feet. Next, rub the curved bottom of the spoon on the bottoms of your feet (in any pattern you wish). This helps activate little energy centers on the bottoms of the feet.

Aim to do this for a few minutes at a time, at least once or twice a day. This is a practice that is beneficial to do all the time, whether you are trying to heal from a major challenge or simply maintain a healthy energy flow.

## 2: Encourage a Crossover Energy Pattern

For optimal functioning of the mind and body, energy should flow in a crossover pattern in the body. This is the body's natural way. Think about how many crossover movements are natural to the body: the brain using both its left and right hemispheres together, our arms swinging across our body when we walk, crawling in a crossover direction when we are babies, and more. Even our DNA is a crossover pattern. If your energy system has become scrambled, it will stop crossing over and start flowing in an up-and-down pattern in your body. In Donna Eden's work, where I first learned about this, it's called a "homolateral" energy flow. When your energy is running in this homolateral pattern, you are not at your full healing capacity. Luckily, the correction for this is easy, as long as you are persistent. Retraining your body's energy to flow in a crossover pattern can be as simple as reminding it to do so—very consistently. Even once you reach your healing goals, this is something that you can continue doing daily. Keeping the crossover energy pattern strong in the body is essential to gain, and maintain, your well-being.

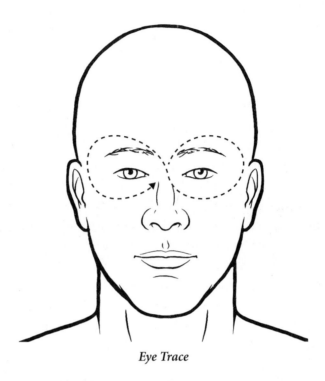

*Eye Trace*

### Trace Around the Eyes

Tracing around the eyes in a crossover pattern is a great energy re-training tool that takes very little effort. I've found this technique to be very helpful. Donna Eden also has her own exercises for this that you may want to explore.

First, place the middle finger of one hand at the bridge of your nose in between your eyes. Next, pressing firmly, trace figure eights around your eyes. Start by dragging your finger up about a half inch around one eyebrow, circling on the forehead around to the outside orbit of your eye, then under your cheekbone and back up to the starting point. Continue the pattern while dragging your finger in the same way around the other side of your eye. You'll want to do this full trace about ten times. Repeat it three times a day or however many times feels doable for you.

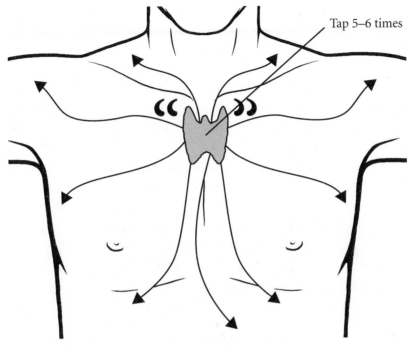

Tap 5–6 times

*Thymus Gland*

### 3: Balance Your Thymus Gland

The thymus gland is the master gland of the body's immune system and is located in the upper part of the chest, behind the breastbone. It sits right over the heart. Because of its location, Dr. John Diamond, a pioneer in the field of holistic healing, says the thymus serves as the link between mind and body.[7] It's located in the area of the heart chakra, which you'll be learning more about in chapter 6.

The thymus is responsible for making T-cells, which are vital to healthy function of the immune system, including protection against allergies, autoimmune diseases, and immunodeficiency. I believe this makes the health of this gland essential to achieving complete and permanent healing. The thymus is so powerful, and so connected to

7. John Diamond, MD, "Thymus Gland, The," *John Diamond, MD,*
   www.drjohndiamond.com/qdiamond-wikipediaq/129-thymus-gland-the.

the rest of the body, that almost any block or imbalance in the body, no matter where it is located, can be cleared through balancing it. In chapter 7, you'll learn how to clear stuck emotions from your body using the thymus gland.

### Tap Your Thymus

Tapping the thymus gland using your fingertips acts as a stimulating, strengthening, and balancing exercise. It's quick and of great benefit to your overall system. Simply tap for about 15–30 seconds while you breathe deeply. This should be done at least three times a day. To make it easy to integrate, you can tie this exercise to other daily activities like getting a drink of water or going to the bathroom. Make a habit of doing thymus tapping each time you do the other activity.

Your thymus gland might be tender when you tap. Do not stop because of this. Tenderness is usually a sign that there is some stagnant energy there, which means you really need this exercise. Over time, as it becomes more balanced, it will become less sore.

## 4: Inch Your Way to Better Thoughts and Feelings

If you have been interested in spirituality for any time at all, you are most likely familiar with the law of attraction. This is often called "The Secret," made popular by the movie with the same name. The law of attraction is based on the idea that "like attracts like." This means that we attract or draw to us whatever energy we are putting out there. While the concept of the law of attraction is wonderful, we have a tendency to place blame on ourselves when things aren't working right. Also, people often make the mistake of trying to force drastic change while they are already in a place of great struggle. This is rarely successful and can even backfire, creating a situation where you end up more frustrated, fighting against what is even harder. I'm determined to help you develop a new and positive experience with this process. I know just how powerful it can be! Instead of too-grand attempts, here we will learn just how effective baby steps can be.

## The Basic Concept: Whatever You Focus On Grows

We know now that our bodies, like the universe, are full of vibrational frequencies. The law of attraction, which is based on energy and vibration, states, "That which is like unto itself is drawn." It means that we are all sending signals out like antennae, picking up on and drawing back to us exactly what we are tuned in to. Similar vibrational frequencies attract each other. Some examples are: frequencies of love attract more love; frequencies of fear attract more experiences that cause fear; frequencies of lack (whether it be linked to money, love, or health) attract more lack.

In other words, whatever vibration or energy you give attention to in your life is drawn back to you from this big universal pool, or what Pam Grout, author of *E-Squared* and *E-Cubed*, calls the "field of infinite potentiality." No matter what you call the energy force, though, we are saying that whatever you focus your energy on grows. So if you are feeling really good and full of positive emotions, you are sending out that signal to the Big U, drawing "matches" for that, such as health, abundance, and love, back to you. If you are feeling bad and are full of yucky emotions, you are sending that signal out and are drawing more of what matches that, such as lack, poverty, illness, and negativity. As we learned in the section on surrender, it's important to be okay with where you are. What's really cool is this: It's much easier to be okay with where you are if you shift your thinking about where you are to a more positive place. And if you shift your thinking about where you are to a more positive place, you'll then attract more of that positive vibration, which will help you move forward.

When I first learned about the law of attraction, it scared the bejeezus out of me and I hated the concept. I worried that every negative thought was making me sick. I decided I'd just pretend it never existed and I'd be just fine. But in time, I got my first law-of-attraction slap in the face when I attended a healing conference. Someone was giving an example about healing from cancer and, on a whim, asked the audience members if those with cancer would raise their hands. When the hands went up in the 500-plus-person crowd, it became obvious that

95 percent of those with cancer were seated next to each other in one long row of chairs. Astoundingly, after a short discussion, the row of people admitted almost none of them knew each other or that their seatmates had cancer. They had just been drawn together. *Hello, law of attraction*, right?

This is when I realized that hating the law of attraction and ignoring it is much like playing a game without reading the rules. So I decided to look at it again, in a different way, and find a way to make it work for me. When I did, I was able to be less terrified and more empowered by it. I truly believe it helped me feel better in my everyday struggle to be okay with what I was living through. Not only that, but I do believe it helped me heal, too. That's why I really want to help you understand and use it—without any of the bad feelings or fear I had.

Let me reassure you here that all of the work you will be doing throughout this book will increase your vibration, your positive energy, and help you shift your thoughts, and therefore will automatically work to your benefit regarding the law of attraction. The less negative energy you are storing within your body, the higher your overall vibration and energetic focus will be, without even consciously trying. You're already moving in the right direction just by being here. Hooray! However, changing your conscious thought pattern is something you can do right now, and all the time. That's why I am sharing this process with you here.

## My Perspective on the Law of Attraction

Because of the "like attracts like" concept, the law suggests that by simply changing your thoughts, you can change how you feel, which then affects your energetic vibration and your reality. Most law-of-attraction gurus teach that your thoughts create your reality—end of story.

I am a bit of a law-of-attraction liberalist, though. I believe our thoughts and the vibrations behind those thoughts greatly influence our reality. Like, big time. We are co-creators in our lives. Nothing happens completely *to* us. However, I think there are some other factors at play, too. As much as I believe that we are powerful beings, I also believe that sometimes yucky things just happen in life, and we can't make ourselves crazy trying to trace back to how we "attracted" them.

As far as shifting your energy to the positive, here's what you need to know. When your desire or vibration aligns completely with your highest good, *that* is your superpowered point of attraction. What that means is that you're in charge of trying to send out the best signal possible (yee-haw!), but the universe is also conspiring for your highest good. Delays in manifestation have always been beneficial for me, so don't jump to the conclusion for yourself that they are due to some wrongdoing or thinking on your part. Your manifestation process has some universal puppet strings attached and they're pulling you in the right direction, too. In other words, you're pretty darn cool and powerful, but it's not 150 percent you, okay?

I know it can be hard to swallow the idea of being in such a powerful co-creating position of our realities, because we have learned that everything in life happens to us. And it can feel like just so much responsibility to know we can change things to such a drastic degree. In her book *A Return to Love*, Marianne Williamson, an author and spiritual leader, says, "Our deepest fear is not that we are inadequate. Our deepest fear is that we are powerful beyond measure. It is our light, not our darkness, that most frightens us." Truth.

In addition to making us afraid of our power, the law of attraction often activates our "blame-brain" mode. *It's my fault for thinking negative thoughts.* Before you start to freak out, though, it's important to remember a couple of key things.

First, manifestation doesn't happen instantly. Hallelujah! The vibration must have some momentum or force behind it. That means that you get lots of time to practice turning your attention to what you want to attract more of and turning away from that which you don't want. Trust me, I have many, many "imperfect" thoughts and I don't immediately get struck down by terrible things. It's because each of my fleeting thoughts does not hold enough power to throw some cosmic force into a fit. Thank goodness.

Another thing to keep in mind is that intention counts for a lot. Having strong intention that we want to feel better or feel relief from our current situation is actually a high vibration. So even when we're feeling really, really crappy, we have the biggest opportunity to use that to send out the signal of *I want to feel good*. We can focus on the positive feeling or desire of the good. Our strong desire to feel good counts for so very much, so even these "bad times" are nothing to beat yourself up about. Great news, right? This Abraham-Hicks quote explains it so well: "There will be a time, not so far from now, that you will look back on this phase of your life and instead of condemning it or beating up on it… Instead of blaming or guilting, you will feel appreciation for it, because you will understand that a renewed desire for life was born out of this time period that will bring you to physical heights that you could not have achieved without the contrast that gave birth to this desire." [8]

Think of the law of attraction as a universal matchmaking service. It's not out to hurt or punish anyone. It's just trying to find an energetic match to and for you. No one gets in trouble for "bad" or "negative" thoughts or beliefs. It's all just an energy dance we are doing with the universe. It's our job to learn to be our best vibration and just let the universe match us up real nice with what's meant to be for us.

## Find a Better-Feeling Focus

Feeling better is really all about a subtle shift from always focusing on what's going wrong to focusing on what's going right, even if there doesn't seem to be much going right. I'm not at all asking you to ignore the negative (trust me, I tried and that definitely doesn't work). But acknowledging it and feeling it and then choosing to shift your thinking and feeling to even just a slightly better focus is a very healing practice. This will help during the times of surrender when you must work with what you have in the moment. For this practice, baby steps are actually preferred. You can inch yourself to feeling good where you are, and it will be much easier than trying to make massive leaps. If you find a

---

8. Abraham-Hicks, "Law of Attraction Journals," *Abraham-Hicks Publications,* www.abraham-hicks.com/lawofattractionsource/journal.php.

way to spin a thought toward the positive even just one time a week, you're headed in the right direction.

### Focus on a Solution

While focusing on symptoms and discontent is going in the wrong direction, focusing on a solution can invoke the positive. It doesn't matter what the *thing* is. As long as you can find a way to feel good about it, your signals are golden. Many of us who are strong believers in the natural healing paradigm can become desperate or down if we turn to anything other than natural healing modalities. We feel like failures. Really, though, any energy you put toward your healing can be beneficial, as long as you find a way to feel good about it. I'll give you this example so you can see how it works, even with something you might tend to feel bad about. Instead of saying or thinking "I'm taking medicine because this virus is destroying my body and I can't heal myself fast enough," you'd shift to "I am taking this medicine to help heal my body while I do the inner work. This is giving me an opportunity to relax and get some support to heal my body, which will help me feel good even faster."

Do you see how that works? Do you see how that would help you relax into where you are right now? Changing your thoughts and focus can be done in a subtle way and still be powerful. Your next thoughts could be something like "I won't need this support forever." "I'm thankful I have this option so I can relax because that's healing." "It feels good that it's not all on me right now."

This type of thought-pattern transformation helps you find relief with where you are, and in that, you raise your vibration, too. Remember the surrender experience we talked about earlier? Well, the gentle redirection of your thoughts fits right into that. The fastest way to get to a new, better-feeling situation is to make peace with your current situation. If you constantly fight against the unfairness of your situation, you hold yourself as a match to that energy, and it's very hard to get somewhere better.

### Identify What You Want

Stop when you find yourself talking about or thinking about what you *don't* want, and immediately start telling yourself what you *do* want. Instead of "I can't stand this pain anymore. I can't live like this because it's just so horrible," try "I want to feel good. I want to be able to live freely." Do not use any negative words when you shift your talk, because whatever you focus on grows. You are trying to grow the positive, which is what you *do* want. If you focus on "I don't want to feel this way," you are giving your focus to feelings of what you don't want and sending out signals for that very thing.

### Journaling

I don't keep a journal in the traditional sense. However, I do have a "manifestation journal" that I use occasionally. In it, I write not about how I feel, but how I *want* to feel or what I *want* to be happening. This is an excellent way to raise your vibration and start feeling good about things even if you aren't quite there yet in reality. It invokes the emotion or feeling that you do want. For example, when my literary agent was shopping my work around, I was going through some cycles of self-doubt, which all writers go through. But in my journal, I was actually writing about how good it felt to know I was working with the right publisher and how perfectly everything was working out. I imagined the call I got from my agent and described it in my journal as if it had already happened. By adding details about the call, the offer, and how it made me feel, I was triggering the positive vibration of my desire in an effort to help me manifest that into reality. And we know how influential feeling good is by now, right? For this exercise, just write your journal or diary entry as you would any other, but make it up! Write as if all your grandest desires have come true that day. This technique really is effective, not to mention fun.

### Find the "Why"

By asking yourself why you want something, you can bring up the positive emotion that will help you attract more of it. Remember, thoughts alone are not enough—we need the feeling behind them.

For example, ask yourself, "Why do I want this healthy body?" Your answer may be something like, "So I can travel again." "So I can work full-time doing something I love." "So I can be a part of the family more." Visualizing these things will bring up the positive emotion to shift your vibration to a positive place. Pay attention to how you feel when you're doing this shifting and visualizing. If something feels bad to visualize (even if it's seemingly positive), find something else to focus on that invokes only positive emotion. Our hidden fears and agendas can sometimes bring up negative emotions, so pay careful attention to this.

* * * * * * * *

You now have three very solid ways to turn your attention to a positive place. But before we wrap up, here's one last, but very important, reminder. You are not allowed to use this knowledge as a weapon for blame. I truly believe it's our job to do what we can to hold a positive vibration, but timing is divine and sometimes things are just doing what they need to do because of something we can't see. It's important not to blame ourselves when things don't happen as we intend, but instead to just keep on doing what we can. Keep inching forward. You're doing just great.

You now know some powerful ways to build a strong healing foundation: correcting polarities by grounding, organizing your energies by encouraging a crossover pattern, balancing the thymus gland, and inching your way to better thoughts and feelings. Make sure you attend to them all lovingly and very consistently. This is where it all starts, baby!

In the next chapter, we will learn how to identify blockages so we can really start to balance the energy system for deep healing.

*Part Two*

\* \* \* \* \* \* \* \* \* \* \* \* \* \* \*

# Identify Blockages

I get emails and questions about various energy-therapy techniques from around the world, all amounting to virtually the same thing: "Is this technique effective?" These emails usually include links and summaries and explanations of how each technique works. Sometimes I am familiar with them, and sometimes I'm not. But it doesn't matter, because here's the thing: there are many wonderful and effective techniques out there, and while I have my favorites (which you will learn in part three), the specific techniques you use are less important than you think.

The essential ingredient for your clearing is to make sure you work on the things that are keeping you stuck. A technique has its full power only if you are applying it to something relevant to your challenge. That's why you are going to spend a lot of time learning how to figure out exactly what's connected to your challenges in the first place. In order to align with your healing, I am going to help you identify the blockages that prevent you from doing so. Once you've identified those blockages, we can work on releasing them.

The two best ways I know to identify blockages are by using a technique called *muscle testing* to get answers from the subconscious mind, and by learning to interpret the language of our bodies. Both of these approaches will allow you to view your current challenges in a whole new light. First, you will learn how to ask your subconscious mind, which is like a virtual tape recorder, exactly what you need to work on. Next, you will learn to interpret your body's own language, which can provide major clues for your healing.

Then, when you apply the techniques in this book—and maybe even some others that you already know—you'll be aiming them at the origin of the imbalance. That's the true key to effectiveness. That's where the magic happens.

*Chapter Five*

\* \* \* \* \* \* \* \* \* \* \* \* \* \*

# Get Answers from the Subconscious Mind

*We can't solve problems by using the same kind of thinking we used when we created them.*

—COMMONLY ATTRIBUTED TO ALBERT EINSTEIN

What is keeping me from feeling calm? Why can't I get better? How come this person triggers me with every little word they speak? Why do I sabotage all my efforts to help myself? What is it that makes me so overwhelmed with life? What is contributing to this illness or challenge?

If you recognize any of these questions, you already have the answers; you just haven't been able to access them yet. There is an entire separate part of your being that's really in control of your life—and that's your subconscious mind. The subconscious mind is like a human computer, recording everything that has happened in our lives. This includes programming we receive as children, through memories, messages, perceptions, and experiences. Our subconscious mind then makes "rules" to live by based on that data or programming. The subconscious mind is basically, in kid terms, *the boss of us!*

In this chapter, you'll learn about the programming of the subconscious mind, the importance of tapping into that programming in order to heal, and exactly how to do that using a technique called muscle testing (sometimes called energy testing or applied kinesiology).

For most of my healing journey, I was using my conscious mind to try to unravel my challenges, and I wasn't getting very far at all. When I learned how to access my subconscious mind through the easy process of muscle testing, my healing increased tenfold.

The information I found in my subconscious mind was totally surprising, hugely helpful, and also a little bit crazy. Some of it made no logical sense and shocked me to the core. I soon learned, though, that the emotions are not logical. I never would have linked many of my challenges to the things that they were actually connected to, especially at first. But that was the good news. I suddenly had access to information I had never known about, worked on issues I had never been aware of, and subsequently got results I had never gotten. Now that I've been doing this for a long time, I think of muscle testing as training wheels on a bicycle. So many things come to me naturally now, but muscle testing was the first way I learned to tap into the body's infinite wisdom. When I first learned muscle testing, I felt like I had just been given the equivalent of a never-ending ladder in a child's board game. I'm about to give you that pass too.

The subconscious mind will do anything to protect us or do what it thinks is good for us, according to its rules or programming. In terms of neurological processing tasks, the subconscious mind is more than a million times more powerful than the conscious mind. It's actually pretty awesome how the subconscious mind works because so much of our life is on autopilot. We don't have to think about how to do mundane tasks or bodily functions. It's not so awesome, though, if there are rules in your subconscious mind that strongly oppose everything your positive-thinking conscious mind is trying to attain—like your well-being. Let's be honest. When you're wrestling with something a million times more powerful than you, what will most likely win? In order to change the programming or rules we live and react from, we need to actually identify the rules first.

## The Subconscious Mind Is Programmed

Scientists have discovered that the subconscious controls up to 95 percent of our lives. Only 5 percent of our memories and other data reside in the conscious mind, which leaves that giant 95 percent in charge. You see the predicament here. Our lives are basically being run by the subconscious mind, which is functioning using a set of rules that were created during early childhood. When you find out exactly what these rules in your subconscious mind are, you will see why you've been stuck for so long.

Getting answers from your subconscious mind is essential to your healing because you can't change what you aren't aware of. And, if you're anything like I was or like many of my clients are, you aren't aware of most of the things that desperately need to be changed so that you can heal.

For instance, you might feel like anger is causing a huge stress on your body and you might contribute your anger issues to, say, your mother. Oh, how we love to blame our mothers, right? However, that is your logical mind and its reasoning putting that together for you. Your mother issues might not be your mother issues at all, but with only your current knowledge, you could spend years working on them from that angle. In essence, you'd be chasing the wrong train and not have any clue. I often see clients who have been going to therapy for twenty years working on something like anger at their mother, only to find out later, through connecting to their subconscious mind, that their challenges are linked to something completely different, like a classmate in second grade who called them names. This is often surprising, but true! When they clear the energy imbalances connected to that, change happens.

While you may jump to connect your challenges to specific experiences or ages, there is often no logical rhyme or reason for what might actually be connected. I often find that experiences will come up through muscle testing that my client has no conscious connection with. I do tend to see patterns of certain ages and experiences pop up for significant times in people's lives, such as the start of school or a sibling being born. The actual experience may seem insignificant now, but a lot of how an experience affects us is connected to our capacity to handle it and process it at the specific age it happened.

I'll show you what I mean in this example. When Emily came to me to clear the energy behind daily panic attacks, she told me she had always connected them with her parents' divorce at age ten. However, as we worked with muscle testing, as you'll learn to do shortly, we learned that this issue was actually tied to age three. The only thing she remembered happening at that time was that her uncle moved from across the street to a neighborhood about fifteen minutes away. Now, to our adult brains, that seems like no big deal, right? And Emily still saw her uncle very often. But at age three, it is huge if your best friend and a source of security is no longer a daily presence. Perhaps that was the original source of the panic that got retriggered later when her dad moved out of the house during her parents' divorce. The original experience or event could be seemingly small in the larger scope of her life, but the age or time in her life was a big influencer in how it affected her.

## Access Your Subconscious Mind with Muscle Testing

Let's talk about how this testing works, and more importantly, how this can get you to your next level of healing.

There is just one basic concept you need to understand before I can teach you how to get answers from the subconscious mind. As you know now, the body has within it and surrounding it an electrical network or grid, which is pure energy. This encompasses the energetic interaction between our physical body and our subconscious mind. Our nervous system is like a very long antenna, picking up on energetic frequencies that directly affect our body—energies too subtle for even scientific instruments to measure. That electrical system, which is connected to your subconscious mind, responds to both positive and negative influences or energies. If anything impacts your electrical system that does not maintain or enhance your body's balance (in other words, it doesn't feel good to your body), your body's energy flow will temporarily "short-circuit," affecting the energy running through your muscles. Things that might have an impact on your electrical system are thoughts, emotions, foods, and other substances.

In order to find out what your subconscious mind and body are congruent with, or "agree" with, we can ask them questions directly. We'll then decipher the answers depending on the response of your body's muscles to those questions (hence the term muscle testing).

If we make a statement that your body and your subconscious resonate with, your electrical system will continue to flow and the circuits will remain strong, allowing your muscles to retain strength. If we make a statement that your subconscious mind considers false, your energy system will temporarily short-circuit and your body (muscles) will quickly react by weakening or locking up.

Each of those reactions will give us a way to read what your body is saying. It's simply a really cool way we can ask your body questions and get clear answers—like a telephone to the subconscious mind.

## Two Ways to Muscle-Test
### The Standing Test (Muscle Testing)

One way of muscle testing that is typically easy for beginners to learn is called the Standing Test. It works on the following basis. Your thoughts and emotions produce a certain response in your nervous system, which is connected to your brain, affecting your motor response (movement of your body). The unconscious part of you that isn't relying on logic and rational thought will naturally be drawn to something it sees as positive or the truth, and will naturally be repelled by something that it doesn't read as truthful for you.

If you ask questions when your body is in a relaxed but standing position (but still able to move without obstruction), you will involuntarily sway—either slightly backward or slightly forward—which will help you decipher if your body agrees with something you say or rejects it. Remember, words are really just energy.

If you have trouble standing, this can be done in a chair. Through this technique, we are essentially using the body as a pendulum.

To make sure your energy is balanced, which is an important part of accurate muscle testing, you're going to perform the Thymus Tap and Eye Tracing exercises from chapter 4. This exercise will help ensure that your energy isn't scrambled and can also be used as a quick energy-balancing tool.

Stand or sit up straight with your feet about shoulder-width apart, pointing directly forward. Ensure both feet are directly forward and neither is slightly turned in or out. Relax your body, with your hands down at your sides. Close your eyes if you are able to stand safely with your eyes closed. Take a big, deep breath.

Now you are ready to ask your body some questions. Your energy system will be picking up on the energy of what you are saying and reacting to the questions involuntarily.

First, you're going to make sure you get an accurate base test. This is just to make sure your body is responding properly so you can trust the rest of the testing and know it's accurate.

Say this statement out loud: *Show me a yes.* Your body should involuntary tip slightly forward, meaning "yes." It is showing you that it's in agreement or in resonance with what you are saying. Next, say this statement out loud: *Show me a no.* Your body should involuntary tip slightly backward, meaning "no." It is showing you that it is rejecting or is repelled by what you're saying.

Alternatively, you can do a base test using your name. Say this statement out loud: *My name is _____.* Your body should involuntary tip slightly forward, meaning "yes." It is showing you that it's in agreement or in resonance with what you are saying.

Next, say this statement out loud: *My name is frog.* Your body should involuntary tip slightly backward, meaning "no." It is showing you that it is rejecting or is repelled by what you're saying.

You might experience some personal variations to the standard forward or backward responses. For example, I have a few clients who kind of swing and lean to the left for "yes" and stay pretty neutral for "no." We figured out this was just their body's own variation and we embraced it. We get accurate answers now that we know exactly how their body gives us a yes or no. Be open to your own variations, too.

If you are getting the total opposite responses to what you should (meaning backward for "yes" and forward for "no), it is most likely because your energy is not balanced enough. Repeat the Thymus Tap and Eye Tracing exercises, take a few deep breaths, and relax. It would also be very beneficial to do a grounding exercise. Being too cerebral interferes with the process of letting your body respond naturally. You'll get it. Just keep trying.

Let's play around with this technique just a little bit more now so you can see how helpful it can be.

Say this statement out loud and notice your body's response: *It is 100 percent safe for me to heal.* Alternatively, you can ask it in question form and notice your body's response: *Is it 100 percent safe for me to heal?* The format you use to ask the question has no bearing on how your body responds, so choose whatever feels more natural to you— either a question or a statement.

Just relax and let your body either "sway" forward gently or sway backward gently, which is how it will answer you. This will happen without you consciously doing anything. Your only job is to relax enough to let it happen. If your body pulls slightly forward, your subconscious mind and body are essentially saying "yes," meaning you are in alignment with that question or statement. You do, at a core level, believe it's safe for you to heal. You agree with it at a subconscious level. That's excellent.

If your body tips or pulls backward, moving away from the statement, your subconscious mind and body are saying "no," it's not safe for you to heal. Don't be alarmed, though. That answer is actually the norm, and new information can help you. You'll be learning how to clear this belief, along with lots of other beliefs that might be blocking you, later in chapter 8. We need your body to agree at a core level that it's safe for you to heal, or your supersmart subconscious mind will do everything in its almighty power to keep you from healing.

When muscle testing, you need to relax, detach from the outcome or answer, and focus only on the question. Because your body will respond to the energy of thoughts, emotions, and more, you want to make sure you are focusing only on the issue you want answers about. It's human nature to want to analyze and resist what doesn't make sense, but if you can really let go and stay open, this tool will change your life.

Now let's use this same testing for another purpose: to see how bringing a stressor to mind affects your energy system. Get in your muscle-testing position. Check to make sure your feet are pointing forward and then close your eyes. Think of something negative, such as the break-up of a relationship, a fight you had with someone, a fear you have, or a time when you were belittled by your boss. Notice if your body sways forward or backward.

Your body will most likely sway slightly backward, which means your electrical system has temporarily short-circuited because that energy is having a stressful or negative impact you.

Now think about what it would be like if that specific stressor was not only introduced into your energy field temporarily but was there all the time—a belief that convinces you that you are unsafe, or an experience from the past that you can't seem to let go of. Your body would constantly be in a state where your energy flow is disrupted and affecting all your tissues, organs, and just the general function of that supercool body you have.

Can you see how, over time, if you don't release these energetic imbalances or your reactions to these stressors, it could take a serious toll on you?

I consider muscle testing to be an energy-detection technique rather than an energy-healing technique, but it's one that is unparalleled to anything else you'll learn because it can give you endless clues as to which experiences, emotions, and beliefs to clear (which we'll be digging into more in part three).

You should be aware that there are many muscle-testing techniques available out there to explore on your own. While the Standing Test is often the easiest to teach, it is important to know that there is much more you can learn on this topic.

### *The Arm Test (Muscle Testing)*

I'm going to share one more muscle-testing method with you quickly. I call this the *Arm Test*. To start, stretch your non-dominant arm out in front of you as if you're reaching for something. Now bend at the elbow so your forearm and hand are at a 45-degree angle. Your palm will be facing out. It will look like you are doing a lazy version of the "stand back" or "stay away from me" hand gesture. Next, take the pointer and middle fingers of your dominant hand and place them just behind the wrist bone (toward the elbow) on your other arm.

Exactly as you did with the Standing Test, you're going to formulate "yes" or "no" statements or ask your body "yes" or "no" questions. After you make the statement or ask the question, you'll use your two fingers to press against the other arm, right behind the wrist (toward the elbow). You want to use only about two pounds of pressure here (this would be considered a light to medium pressure). Allow your non-dominant arm to resist slightly without fighting. When you press with your two fingers, after verbalizing the question or statement, you're going to gauge your body's response to figure out what answer your subconscious is giving you.

When we did the Standing Test, tipping forward was your body's "yes" response and tipping backward was your body's "no." With the Arm Test, your body is saying "yes" or "I'm in resonance" with the question or statement when your arm has no problem resisting the gentle pressure of those two fingers (your arm stays strong). This means that you do not feel any "give" in the arm. If your arm feels like it loses a bit of strength and wants to give way under the pressure, your muscle is temporarily short-circuiting, like we talked about at the beginning of this chapter. Your body is saying "no" or "I'm not in resonance" with the question or statement.

Muscle testing is not a fight between your two arms. You are simply noticing if your non-dominant arm weakens with the slight pressure from your two fingers. The key is not to make your non-dominant arm too rigid and not to press too hard or lightly with your two fingers. It's like getting the flame on a gas stove just right. You'll find the sweet spot that works for you.

If you have trouble performing the Standing Test and the Arm Test, even after lots of practice, I encourage you to discover and learn other self-testing techniques until you find a fit for you. I can't stress enough the value of this technique. I almost gave up on it out of frustration when I couldn't get the hang of it at first, which would have caused a delay in my healing.

The following examples will give you a sneak peek of the types of blocks that you'll be able to detect for yourself with muscle testing. I'll be walking you through exactly how to do this for yourself in part three, but for now, I just want to give you a quick glimpse into the world you are going to open up to.

## Muscle-Testing Example Stories

Tim came to me for help with severe eczema. He itched constantly and had no idea why. He had been to psychotherapists, dermatologists, acupuncturists, and more. As always, I suspected there was an emotional component to this itching. I taught Tim the basics of muscle testing and walked him through several questions.

First, I had Tim ask his body through muscle testing if it believed the itching was beneficial for him in some way. I was testing to see if his body saw this problem as a benefit to him in some way, which is very common. I knew that until we cleared that belief, it would be difficult to clear the itching. We got a "yes" response. I then thought of beliefs, or reasons, his body might have for not wanting to let this go. We asked his body in first person, "Do I need the itching as a distraction from something scary?" Tim's body signaled a "yes." We knew we were on the right track.

As you'll discover in the next chapter, itching is often the body's message for someone or something "getting under your skin." In order to try to find out what or who it was, I asked, "Is this itching linked to a specific age?" Again, it was a "yes." Next, we started testing ages, breaking them down into 20-year periods (ages 0–20, ages 20–40, etc.), knowing his body had the recording of exactly when this energy imbalance began in his system. "Is this itching linked to an age between ages 0–20?" His body let us know the answer was "no." "Is this itching linked to ages 20–40?" We got a "yes" and narrowed it down to the exact age by breaking it down to 10 years, 5 years, then individual years. His body told us through muscle testing that the itching was linked to age 32.

Tim and I talked about what had happened that year and came up with a few ideas. We had an idea of which one was linked to the itching, but suspended judgment. Tim had been working on this issue for quite some time, and I reminded him of the importance of being open to the option that made the least sense, just in case it actually was tied to this. And guess what? It was. Through muscle testing, his body confirmed that the itching was somehow linked to getting fired at age 32.

Here are the questions we asked his body to get to this conclusion. There is no specific formula for what to ask. We were just asking questions that we were wondering about and knew his body would have the answer to. "Is this eczema linked to a family member?" We got a "no." We pressed on: "Is this eczema connected to a past romantic relationship?" Again, a "no." Finally we asked, "Is this eczema linked to career?" We got our "yes." Then we asked, "Is it linked to getting fired from the job?" We got another "yes." This surprised Tim because he'd had a terrible relationship break-up at age 32, but apparently his body had discharged that old energy from his system. Realizing Tim was still allowing that experience to "get under his skin" (he felt he had been fired unfairly), we worked on clearing it using techniques you will be learning in chapter 7.

Tim saw great improvement in the itching in just the first few weeks and continued to improve from there. While there is typically not just one thing contributing to an ongoing problem, you can use this system of asking questions and narrowing down options to clear away all of the layers that might be linked to the challenge or ailment.

In this next session example, I helped a client identify a belief that was acting as a healing block. Ellen was having a very hard time with her self-esteem, which was causing a constant state of stress that was most likely exacerbating her physical symptoms and interfering with her healing process. When we talked about her challenges and the negative self-talk she struggled with, she said sadly, "I know what belief is causing all of this. It always comes down to me not feeling good enough." Instantly we had something to work with.

Here are the questions we had Ellen ask her body: "Is my belief that I'm not good enough related to a specific person?" When we got a "yes" from her body, we continued. "Is it related to Mom?" We got a "no" answer. "Is it related to Dad?" We got a "yes" answer and made a note of it. "Is this belief related to a specific experience from my past?" Through these questions, we were able to gain enough information and insight that Ellen's intuition kicked in and suddenly an idea popped into her head. We double-checked it with her body, asking, "Is the feeling that I'm not good enough linked to Dad yelling at me for not getting an A on

Ms. Black's spelling test?" Yep, there it was—the place where it all had started.

We were excited to have found such an important event that we could then clear for Ellen. We continued on over several sessions, clearing many similar unprocessed experiences being stored in her body, always playing on the "not good enough" belief—all by asking questions that led us to exactly what was contributing to her low self-esteem.

We then used the process you'll learn in chapter 8 for clearing harmful beliefs, such as Ellen's "I'm not good enough." That was the beginning of shifting this pattern for her.

In both of these examples, we were simply asking questions that we might already have been thinking or wondering about. We allowed our curiosity to lead us. We were just putting the questions into a clear, concise format in which we could ask the body.

## Tips for Your Muscle-Testing Practice

Here are some questions you can ask to get some more practice identifying blockages. We are going to cover all of these types of blocks in depth soon, but for now, it's a very curious process to play with. You'll be able to clear the blocks later. So if you come up with any insightful answers, make sure to write them down.

- Is there energy from a specific age in my life that is suppressing my immune system?
- Is there a specific experience from my past causing a stress response in my body?
- Is there a specific organ or gland in my body that is storing unhealthy emotional energy?

Remember, if you pull forward using the Standing Test or your arm stays strong using the Arm Test, all your body is saying is "yes, this is true for me." If that's not working for you, there is no need to panic. We'll be changing things in the next chapter.

Because I had such a difficult time muscle testing at first, I quickly learned all the tricks to make it as accurate as possible. Here are some ideas for you:

- Make statements or ask questions using only affirmative language. This means if you are trying to find out if you believe deep down that you *can* heal, you'd use the statement "I can heal" and see how your body responds, instead of using "I can't heal." It is confusing to the body to use negatives in this way while muscle testing. Another example is using the statement "My liver is functioning properly" instead of "My liver isn't functioning properly."

- Make sure you're hydrated. Electricity requires water, and if you're dehydrated, your electrical system won't be working the way it should, making it difficult to get answers.

- Relax. Relax your body and your mind. Know that any answers you receive will only work toward helping you. There is nothing to be afraid of. I have never uncovered something scary during a session, and neither have my clients. You may have trouble testing if you are feeling doubtful, overthinking, or analyzing the process. I can't emphasize enough just how important it is to let go during this process.

- Ask very clear, concise, and literal questions. The subconscious mind and the body will not interpret questions or statements for their meaning. Use only words that can have only one meaning. For example, it's clearer to ask something like "Is there a specific experience from my past that is preventing me from healing?" rather than "Did something happen to me that's stopping my healing?" The first question is very clear and clean, giving the subconscious mind and the body no reason to be confused in their response.

- Ask questions in different ways. Be creative. Nine times out of ten, altering or clarifying a question will yield a clearer answer. I believe, in part, that sometimes the body won't respond if we're not on the right track or our questions need to be tweaked slightly. Try to incorporate the following words into your questions: component, connected to, related to, triggered by/triggering, harmful, contributing to/contributing, and causing/cause. These are all words that are clear and have no dual meanings. Here are some examples: "Is this back pain connected to a current relationship?" "Is the primary cause of this back pain a belief?" "Is there a person in my life triggering an experience from my past?" (Note: "Triggering" is my favorite phrase to use during muscle testing because it helps us to acknowledge that the present issue may not necessarily be the "real" issue, but rather that something from our past is getting activated by whatever is currently going on in our lives. This means we are getting a two-for-one clearing! We get to release the past and also improve the current issue at hand.)

- Make sure to take a deep breath and pause in between questions to allow your body and brain to recalibrate. Going too fast will cause a sensory overload and your system will freeze up, yielding confusing answers.

- A quick fix, if muscle testing doesn't seem to be working, is to press the fingers of one hand into your bellybutton (this can be over your clothes). Hold them there while you test. This often corrects an energetic flow issue in the body that can make muscle testing difficult.

- Ask the questions slowly and take a few seconds' break in between questions so you don't overload your body. And do not keep repeat-testing the same question. This will overload your circuits and cause your testing to be less accurate. Just learn to trust the answer you get.

- Cautions: Do not use this testing technique to try to predict the future, win the lottery, make major life decisions based on your answer alone, or test yourself for medical diagnoses. None of the answers will be accurate—I and many other very proficient muscle testers can tell you that from experience! Generally speaking, the more attached you are to the answer, the less accurate the testing might be. We are simply using this as a tool to see what our bodies resonate with so we can change anything no longer serving us. Also, move away from electronics (remove your cell phone from your pocket if it's on your body, or move away from your computer). They can interfere with your body's energetic flow.

Again, you'll have lots of opportunities coming up to practice this new skill. I teach it to all new clients, and while most are uncomfortable and untrusting at first, they are eventually glad I made them work through it. You don't need to employ muscle testing to use the healing approach in this book, but it will very likely open you up to brand-new things that would be much harder to access without it.

*Tip:* Throughout this book, I teach you how to clear certain types of imbalances with specific techniques. That's the most effective way to learn. But the truth is that almost any technique can clear almost any challenge. The techniques are widely interchangeable and flexible. Once you've gone through this whole book and understand all the concepts and techniques, you will be able to use your muscle testing to determine which techniques are most beneficial for you in various circumstances. I will teach you how to do this in chapter 11.

You now understand the basics of muscle testing. In part three, I will guide you through using muscle testing to help you find and clear emotional energies that are getting in your way. Learning to understand your body's language is a very different but truly effective way to gain even more knowledge. We're going to dig into that in the next chapter. You'll then be able to use both muscle testing and reading your body's language as a powerful combination to gain more insight for your healing.

*Chapter Six*

\* \* \* \* \* \* \* \* \* \* \* \* \* \*

# Learn the Language
# of Your Body

*The body is honest.*

—SAORI MINOTA

Your body is smart. Like, kind of genius actually. It is talking to you all the time, sending you clues and messages through its symptoms. In a 2012 *Huffington Post* article, Deepak Chopra wrote, "Modern medicine, for all its advances, knows less than 10 percent of what your body knows instinctively."[9] I credit a huge part of my own healing success, and that of my clients, to finding what messages the body is trying to communicate through symptoms. These symptoms are actually metaphors for what's going on internally, on an emotional and energetic level.

Even though I don't have any long-term health issues anymore, I still interpret any temporary symptoms that arise for me. *Is this headache that just popped up trying to get my attention? Does my tummy feel queasy because of something I'm not stopping to deal with?* By becoming aware of this connection, I know I will never again get to a place of *oh my goodness, how did this horrible condition completely sneak in and take over my life?*

In this chapter, I'm going to give you a brand-new way to look at symptoms. You are going to see the body through a lens that offers clues, messages, and metaphors to further your healing. I'll give you

---

9. Deepak Chopra, "The Real Secret to Staying Healthy For Life," *The Huffington Post*, July 30, 2012, www.huffingtonpost.com/deepak-chopra/healthy-lifestyle _b_1694029.html.

real-life examples so you can begin to practice thinking in this way by yourself. I will also provide you with my interpretations of the body's symptoms and its messages. Each condition, symptom, and reaction is a metaphor for some bigger meaning—one that can be used as a clue while you work your way through this book.

Learning the language of the body is an insanely valuable technique, because if you are open to it, you'll start seeing the metaphors in everything. And those can be translated into messages your body is trying to deliver, beliefs your body is holding, old unprocessed experiences you need to let go of, and more. These are all things that you will learn how to clear in part three.

Symptoms are your body's emotional guidance system, which is hard to ignore, resist, or dismiss. I used to become annoyed at my body for always being symptomatic, but in hindsight, I see it was the only completely honest source of information in my life. It called me out—very often. As I became more apt and able to ignore it, it became stronger and louder. It never gave up and didn't cower at my rebellion. It just kept delivering the messages.

After a while, you will become familiar with how your body speaks to you. We each have what I like to refer to as *the loudest link* (my more positive version of the term *the weakest link*). This part (or parts) of your body may feel like your worst enemy, but, in fact, it is your best friend. It'll be the part that acts up first to tell you something is not right. For me, the loudest link is my uterus. If I am not paying attention to something, my uterus will tell me. Another person may have a lower back that goes out when they need a message. Yet another may have a random eye twitch or rash. Another may experience migraines. You get the idea.

## Connect with Your Body

While gently analyzing symptoms, always remember that your body is doing its very best. These messages (symptoms) are being sent with love and helpfulness. Directly connecting with your body in loving and reassuring ways is a worthwhile approach when you want your body to heal.

Here are a few methods of communicating with my body that have been successful for me.

### A Thank-You Prayer

This prayer to my body is one I wrote to help myself connect with it on a healthy level, even through the frustration I often felt because of symptoms. I offer it to you here in the hope that it will bring you some peace, too.

> *Blessed is my body and soul that carries the weight*
> *of a million lifetimes—and remains, anyway.*
> *I thank you for surviving each day, up until now,*
> *And for the ones that will come after this.*
> *I release all resentment of you.*
> *I release all criticism.*
> *I choose to listen to you without judgment.*
> *I choose to let you know I love you.*
> *I choose to allow you to simply be.*
> *Thank you and it is done!*

### Speak Lovingly to Your Body

Sometimes, during periods of horrific menstrual pain, I could do nothing but put my hands over my lower abdomen and talk to my uterus. I'd say aloud that I understood it was trying to tell me something and that I was doing my best to hear what that was. I would make pacts for hot baths and other treats if only "we" could pull it together enough so I could walk to the bathroom without being doubled over. In some very strange way, it helped me connect with my rebellious organ and find love and compassion for all of myself. Talking in a loving way to your body is a useful daily practice for healing.

Sit quietly with your hands over the part of you that needs the most love. Now talk to it, breathe through it, or just send love or compassion to it. It's amazing what being connected to even the parts of ourselves that we're not too happy with at the moment can do for our healing.

*Use Sticky Notes*

I'm a little obsessed with sticky notes. I have them everywhere with reminders and favorite quotes. I also use them for healing. Remember how words are just energy? Writing words or phrases like "I love you," "healing," "strong," or "happy" and putting them in your pockets or on your body can have a healing effect.

Try it. You might just end up following in my footsteps as the "sticky note queen."

*Move and Direct Energy*

Paying special attention to the specific body part in need of healing can be very beneficial. By focusing on the challenged area, organ, gland, or body part in a positive way, you can clear out stagnant energy. You can do this in any way that feels good to you, but here are a few suggestions:

- Tap, stretch, or rub directly on the challenged area. This will help create movement and a healthy flow of energy there.
- Imagine that area of the body bathed in light. Different colors have different frequencies, but the colors of violet, indigo (a color between blue and violet), and blue have some of the highest frequencies, which make them powerful for healing.

Now that you have some positive practices for connecting with your body, you're in a better place to really communicate with it. We're ready to look at what it might be saying.

## Examples of Symptoms as Helpful Clues

When I was writing this book, my menstrual cycles continued as usual, without the excruciating pain I was once shackled by. However, they suddenly became extremely heavy and relentless. Even though my uterus used to send messages in the form of pain, my uterus is still my body's main messenger. Same messenger, but new message. Just to be safe, I checked in with my naturopath, who confirmed that everything, including my hormone levels, was normal. She casually said she believes that sometimes there's just a "spiritual barnacle" of something left that's finally ready to be dealt with. So I took that and ran. My menstrual cycle made me feel like I was "bleeding out," so I thought about that. In what ways in my life did I feel like I was bleeding out? Of course, it hit me! While writing this book, I didn't cut back on my client load; I just added the hundreds of extra hours into my schedule without lightening my burden in any other way. It was so pre-healthy "old me." I felt like I was an output machine with little time for recharge.

When I realized this, I began clearing the beliefs that made me think I had to do it all. I cleared fears about letting my clients down if I took some time off. I took a few weeks off work to focus solely on writing. By not allowing time and space for my creative expression in the way that I needed, I had been suppressing energy in my sacral (second) chakra (governing the uterus), which you will learn about in more detail later in this chapter. I also explored and cleared some resistances to being vulnerable in personal relationships. It is not something I've ever been naturally good at, and it was hindering me at that time in my life more than ever. The second chakra is related to feelings, so this made a lot of sense in relationship to that time in my life.

I didn't beat myself up. I just went through the process of exploring and clearing, knowing that when my uterus was convinced I had gotten the message, it would relax again. And it did. The heavy bleeding subsided after that. Just a few more "spiritual barnacles," I suppose!

Another example of how our body sends us messages comes from a friend I worked with. Amelia couldn't move her neck in either direction more than about fifteen degrees. I asked her when it started and she said just a few years ago. Of course, I then asked her what was going on at that time in her life. She talked a lot about her brother and his wife and how she disapproved of how they were disciplining their children. Amelia didn't have kids herself but definitely had ideas about the "right" and "wrong" ways to raise kids. The neck is a very flexible part of our body, and if we decide to be "stiff" or narrow-minded about something, our necks will often show us what's not working in our lives, through symptoms. We did some clearing on her not being able to allow her brother to take his own direction with his children. We released her fears about him doing it "wrong," and resistance to being flexible in her relationship with her brother's wife. Immediately she could turn her neck to each side about thirty degrees—already a huge improvement.

Based on that initial improvement, I knew there was more to clear, and I had another question pop into my mind. I asked her, if she wasn't so distracted by what her brother and his wife were doing, what would she be focusing on? She immediately said, "Dancing! I used to go to dance class all the time, but my neck won't let me now." Together, we discovered some fears she had about getting back into her passion, which, ironically, was being reinforced by her just being too upset and in pain to do anyway (funny how that works, right?). We worked on those fears, and what do you know, she could immediately turn her head about 50 percent farther on each side! We worked from these two angles over just a couple of sessions and she regained full movement in her neck.

Her neck pain and immobility might have been metaphors for some of these things: fear around dancing and her self-expression, an inability to be flexible in her thoughts and relationships, and the "pain in the neck" she was allowing her brother and wife to be in her life, just by them being themselves. One symptom can be sending several messages, but if you simply explore whatever comes to mind, you'll definitely have some solid ground to work on.

Note: It's very important to understand something here. We are in no way denying the existence of any medical or psychological condition. We are simply looking at a much bigger, holistic picture of your body and working to address any emotional imbalances that might have contributed to the issues in the first place. We are, in essence, asking the body, "Why has this issue manifested here?" "Why has this issue manifested now?" We are trying to use the body's language to get answers that will help you heal. Furthermore, by releasing any extra emotional "burden" from your system, even if not directly related to the condition, your body will have more energy and strength to heal itself. This process is all about doing what we can to minimize stress on the body and maximize healing potential.

## Common Clues, Messages, and Metaphors

I remember at one point in my own healing, as I started to uncover these messages and metaphors, I thought, *The human body is so interesting. I just wish mine wasn't quite this interesting.* You might feel the same; but as best you can, just try to remember that these symptoms are massive clues that will help you heal.

In my work with clients, I see some common patterns in terms of metaphors, messages, and clues that certain types of conditions or symptoms are connected to. It doesn't matter what name or diagnosis your specific collection of symptoms has been given. It is much more important to look at the area being affected and the possible message behind it.

The lists in the rest of this chapter are grouped according to chakras (a part of the subtle energy body); organs, glands, and other parts of the physical body; systems of the body; and conditions you might be experiencing. For each, I will offer examples of what metaphors your body may be using to get a message across. This is my interpretation based on intuition, personal metaphors, energetic understanding, and experience with clients. My outline will give you a variety of ideas to explore. While this is going to be hugely helpful, please do not close yourself off to coming up with even more ideas. Remain open to what messages your own body is trying to give you.

It is sometimes helpful to look at what was happening in your life just before these messages started to show up (in the year or two before). While it is useful to pay attention to the time before the symptoms began, that period might actually represent an issue that goes back to an event even earlier in your life. For example, let's say you were going through a divorce the year before you started having panic attacks. It may seem that your divorce is the triggering incident, but the emotional energy could be even more closely connected to when your own parents got divorced during your childhood

If, when reading these lists, a particular metaphor resonates with you or something "random" like an old memory or person from your life pops into your head, it's likely a big ol' clue from your subconscious mind saying *pay attention to me!* Stay open to whatever is trying to come up and I promise that you'll see opportunities where you once saw roadblocks.

On a final note, you may see the same symptoms, body system, or concept in various places within these lists with different suggested messages. That's because the energy may show up in more than one place and may also mean a variety of things. Just see what resonates with you and leave the rest.

After these lists, you will find a series of questions to help you explore even further. This will get you to start thinking in terms of clues and messages and will help you have a greater understanding of what energies need to be cleared in part three. You'll probably be referring back to this section often while working through part three, using it as a resource for new ideas and direction, so it may be a good idea to mark the page at the start of the lists so you can easily find it.

### Chakras

Chakras are spinning energy centers in the body. There are seven major chakras throughout the body. Chakras store "old stories" and early patterns in the body. Their energies are directly tied to early childhood programming and conditioning. Each chakra governs different areas of the physical body. Energy imbalances in the chakras often show up as symptoms in the related physical area. By noticing which chakras seem to be imbalanced, and studying the chakra's corresponding organs, glands, and muscles, you'll likely find some new clues to work with.

**Crown (Seventh) Chakra**—The crown chakra covers the top of your head down to your eyes. It symbolizes spirituality and your connection to a higher force or power. It is tied to the energy of knowing you can trust life and that you are being taken care of and guided.
*Physical Coverage:* Top of the brain and pineal gland.
*Focus:* Purpose in life and connection to a higher source.

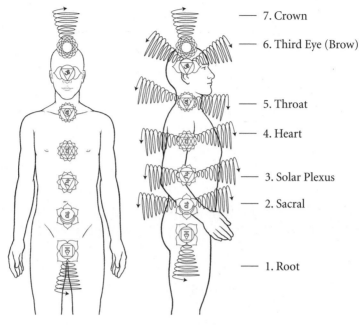

7. Crown

6. Third Eye (Brow)

5. Throat

4. Heart

3. Solar Plexus

2. Sacral

1. Root

*The Seven Chakras*

**Third Eye or Brow (Sixth) Chakra**—The third eye (or brow) chakra is located directly between the eyebrows. It represents intuition, imagination, reflection, and the ability to see things for what or how they are (interpretation). This chakra is responsible for your senses, both sensory and extrasensory perception.

*Physical Coverage:* Eyes, ears, nose, pituitary gland, hypothalamus, skull, and your brain's frontal lobe—considered the emotional control center.

*Focus:* Vision and inner guidance.

**Throat (Fifth) Chakra**—Located in the center of the throat, this chakra is about expression, communication, and truth, both internally and externally. It is the metabolizer of the body, metabolizing information, expression, and more. It is often regarded as the most important chakra of all because it receives information from all the other chakras and processes it, helping to create your unique expression in the world.

*Physical Coverage:* Thyroid gland, throat, tonsils, mouth, and brain stem.

*Focus:* Communication and expression.

**Heart (Fourth) Chakra**—The heart chakra is located in the center of your chest. It is linked to love, intimacy, forgiveness, and the ability to send and receive love. This chakra is also responsible for helping you manifest your heart's desires by sending energetic signals of them out into the world. It spins over your thymus gland, one of the most important glands for the health of your immune system. All emotional conflict can affect heart chakra energy.

*Physical Coverage:* Heart, thymus gland, lungs, upper rib cage and vertebrae, shoulders, arms, and breasts.

*Focus:* Love, relationships, and inner healing.

**Solar Plexus (Third) Chakra**—The solar plexus chakra, located just below the sternum, governs your sense of personal power, including your personal choices and actions in the world. Its energy is tied to self-confidence, self-esteem, and the feeling of having power over your own life. It stores your judgments and opinions about yourself and the world. This chakra is closely linked to your ego and identity and how you relate to the world—who you are in it, what you desire in it, and how you can manifest those desires.

*Physical Coverage:* Kidneys, liver, adrenal glands, pancreas, spleen, stomach, gallbladder, and lower rib cage.

*Focus:* Personal power and positive mentality.

**Sacral (Second) Chakra**—The sacral chakra is located behind the navel in the pelvis. It relates to your joy, creativity, feelings, and childlike qualities. It also represents sexuality. It's tied closely to your stories and conditioning from childhood. This chakra also governs the energy of self-nurturing and self-healing.

*Physical Coverage:* Reproductive organs, bladder, intestines, ileocecal valve (controls and regulates the flow of fecal matter in your body), pelvis, sacrum, and the lumbar region of the spine.

*Focus:* Feelings, joy, and creativity.

**Root (First) Chakra**—The root chakra is located at the base of the spine. It represents your feelings of safety and your primal instinct for survival. It's connected to early childhood beliefs, money, and identity. It deals with abandonment issues, unworthiness, and feeling insecure. It also relates to financial worries at a survival level. This chakra, when healthy, keeps you feeling grounded or rooted in life. What people often describe as "anxiety" is closely linked to root chakra energy imbalance.

*Physical Coverage:* Genitals, legs and feet, and base of spine.

*Focus:* Safety, security, and survival.

### Organs, Glands, and Other Parts of the Body

**Adrenal Glands**—Adrenal glands are part of the endocrine system and are located at the top of the kidneys. They are in charge of producing cortisol. Cortisol is an adrenal hormone, called "the stress hormone," and modulates many of the body's reactions to stress. The adrenals can become fatigued when a person is in a constant state of fear, always feeling on edge or like the other shoe is about to drop. Adrenal glands are dominated by the triple warmer meridian, which is responsible for the fight, flight, or freeze pattern. General stress and feeling like you need to be defended will affect the adrenals.

Adrenal glands are also related to your ability to manage your energy in a healthy way. Being unable to say no and having fears around disappointing others will affect the adrenals. The adrenals can be suppressed by feeling undeserving and feeling lost in relationship to what direction to take in life. Weakened adrenals can be linked to despair and feelings of "what's the point?"

Weakened adrenal glands can show up as problems with the left knee or low back. What people refer to as "anxiety" can be closely related to imbalances of the adrenal glands. Because adrenal glands are part of the endocrine system, their energies and imbalances can affect the thyroid and the reproductive system as well.

*Tip:* Refer to the solar plexus (third) and root (first) chakras for more.

**Arms and Hands**—Arms and hands can be metaphors for carrying too much for others, feeling like your hands are tied in a particular situation, like things are too much or too hot to handle, fear about letting go, holding on too tightly, grasping at straws, difficulty giving and receiving, feeling like you are holding everything together on your own, and fear about things being out of your hands.

*Tip:* Refer to the heart (fourth) chakra for more.

**Back**—Energy affecting your back can be showing you patterns of carrying everything on your back, being unable to stand up for yourself, being stabbed in the back, being afraid to turn your back, turning your back on someone (guilt), turning your back to something scary, living in the past (feeling like it's behind you or following you), wishing you could go back and change something, being afraid that your past (all that stuff "back there") will catch up with you, being unable to back away from a situation, feeling scared to stand up for yourself, and having no backbone with others.

The lower back (root chakra) is usually linked to survival energy, such as family, personal safety, finances/money, and early childhood; the mid-back (solar plexus chakra) is often associated with guilt; and the upper back (heart chakra) may be a metaphor for feeling unsupported.

Imbalanced kidneys can also lead to back pain (particularly low and middle), so it's worth looking at aspects of fear, the primary emotion of the kidneys. Additionally, back discomfort can be connected to the bladder, reproductive organs, small intestine, and large intestine (colon).

*Tip:* Refer to the root (first) chakra, solar plexus (third) chakra, and heart (fourth) chakra for more.

**Bladder**—Bladder issues are often linked to fear and nervousness, being pissed off, or feeling insecure and unsure (wishy-washy). The bladder is connected to the nervous system, energetically. If the nervous system is imbalanced due to stress reactions, it can greatly affect the bladder (a "nervous bladder"). Always feeling on edge or on the fence about something can also irritate the bladder. Situations where we are constantly planning on how to approach someone or something can keep us suspended in nervousness. Imbalances in bladder energy can show up in the lower back, knees, and feet.

*Tip:* Refer to the sacral (second) chakra for more.

**Brain/Head**—Metaphors for this area can be linked to feeling dizzy with anger or fear, being hot-headed, spinning with confusion, feeling like your world has been rocked, feeling overwhelmed, being unable to clear your head, being a headstrong person, being overwhelmed, being clouded, feeling like you can't stop thinking about something or can't get your head around something. Are you "doing your head in" by ruminating over the same worry or thought?

Your head is also linked to feeling connected to a higher source (God, the universe, the Divine) and your spiritual self. Not being able to trust life's flow can create physical symptoms in this area.

Self-criticism and over-thinking are also messages sent by symptoms in the head. Migraines are a common sign of being too hard on oneself.

Headaches and dizziness are associated with the liver meridian's energy, so looking at emotions that affect the liver may also be helpful. These are anger (self-directed or otherwise), resentment, bitterness, and frustration. Sometimes headaches can be linked to sexual fears and experiences or criticism.

Dizziness is linked to the nervous system energetically, which is governed by the bladder meridian. As I mentioned when discussing the bladder, that energy can be linked to nervousness, anger, feeling insecure, and more.

*Tip:* Refer to the crown (seventh) chakra for more.

**Breasts**—Messages that show up in the breasts most often relate to self-nurturing. This might be a message that you are ignoring your own needs. Symptoms in the breasts are often indicators of an inability to turn inward and take care of yourself first. The stomach meridian, or energy pathway, runs directly through the breasts. Because the emotion of worry is linked to the stomach meridian, energy around worry is something to pay attention to.

Because of their location, breasts can be affected by anything that is unresolved in the lungs and heart, including unprocessed grief, inner conflict, and relationships about which you don't have a feeling of inner peace.

*Tip:* Refer to the heart (fourth) chakra for more.

**Cheeks/Sinuses**—Sinus issues can be messages of being congested with old ideas, irritation, or old grief (unreleased tears and snot) or being "stuffed" full of worry. This can also be about feeling stuck in life, without the movement and flow you desire.

The sinuses are connected energetically to your stomach, which relates to the emotion of worry. Many people who have sinus issues also have stomach challenges, and vice versa.

*Tip:* Refer to the third eye (sixth) chakra for more.

**Chest and Lungs**—Symptoms that show up in the chest might have the message of carrying a burden on your chest, having a heavy heart, fear of having an open heart, being in a suffocating situation, or being unable to get something off your chest. (As you can see, many of these are heart-related matters.)

Energy imbalances in the chest area are often linked to energies such as heaviness, grief, depression, rejection, and confusion.

*Tip:* Refer to the heart (fourth) chakra for more.

**Ears**—Ears can be offering metaphors for not being willing or able to hear the truth, listen to yourself, or listen to others; being hurt by the words of another; or being overly sensitive to what others say in general.

Ears are energetically connected to the kidney meridian. Emotions associated with the kidneys are fear, dread, and blaming and are all worth exploring.

*Tip:* Refer to the throat (fifth chakra) for more.

**Eyes**—Metaphors concerning the eyes might deal with clarity and inner knowing. They might include an inability to see the truth, not liking what you see in your own life, not wanting to see what's ahead, refusing to look at the truth, an inability to look forward, not trusting life and the future, or not being able to trust your inner eye or intuition. The kidneys are also linked to the eyes energetically. Emotions associated with the kidneys are fear, dread, and blaming, so it would be interesting to see if those might fit for you too.

Migraines that affect the eyes specifically can be linked to conflict with the inner voice and fear of listening to intuition (which comes from the third eye area, right between your eyebrows). If the issue with the eyes involves dry eyes, this is often linked to fear, nervousness, or inability to show emotion, fear of letting go, and an imbalance in the nervous system. Twitching of the eye (or any other body part, in fact) is energetically linked to the nervous system as well.

*Tip:* Refer to the third eye (sixth) chakra for more.

**Gallbladder**—Your gallbladder secretes bile to help you digest fat and is an important part of your digestive process. It is imbalanced by emotions such as resentment, frustration, guilt, and indecisiveness. If it is a problem, there may be some "fat" or "waste" in your life that you are just not letting go of. Gallbladder imbalance will often result in right knee pain and right shoulder pain.

*Tip:* Refer to the solar plexus (third) chakra for more.

**Heart**—Your heart is a muscle that pumps blood through your entire body, but it is essential to your emotional health as well. According to the Institute of Heart Math, the heart and brain have a continuous two-way dialogue, each affecting the functioning of the other. The signals that go from the heart to the brain can influence emotional and cognitive functioning. The heart is often called the "second brain" of the body and is connected to giving and receiving love and the ability to manifest. It is affected by feelings such as insecurity, abandonment, betrayal, and extending yourself to others but not receiving anything back.

Imbalances or conflicts in the heart often cause dizziness, so this is something else to consider. Insomnia or other sleep challenges are almost always related to matters of the heart, such as inner conflict, feeling unsettled, feeling lost, and not listening to your heart. Unresolved emotional energy in the heart can radiate and affect the shoulders, chest, and neck (including the thyroid).

*Tip:* Refer to the heart (fourth) chakra for more.

**Hips**—Your hips help to lead you forward in life. They also support your lower body. When you are feeling fearful about a new direction in your life or being able to support yourself, it can show up in your hips. Imbalances in the large intestine (colon) can also manifest as pain or discomfort in the hips. Your large intestine is linked to "letting go," so if there is fear about letting go and moving forward, this would be beneficial to address. Imbalances in the uterus or other areas of the reproductive system can also affect the hips.

*Tip:* Refer to the root (first) chakra for more.

**Kidneys**—Your kidneys cleanse your blood and are a large reservoir for your energy. They are imbalanced by emotions such as fear, dread, or feeling unsupported or conflicted. The kidney meridian runs through your feet and legs, so fear around moving forward or stepping out on your own may fit. In Chinese medicine, the kidney energy stores your life force energy and is extremely important. Anything that drains your kidney energy (most often fear) will affect your entire body. Kidney imbalance can also show up as pain or discomfort in your lower and mid back.

*Tip:* Refer to the solar plexus (third) chakra for more.

**Legs, Knees, and Feet**—Challenges with legs and feet can indicate feeling unsafe moving forward, being ungrounded, being unsure of your next step, feeling stuck in the mud, being too fearful to move, feeling like you're sinking, carrying too much emotional weight, being unable to walk away from something, having to walk away from something, and feeling lost/wandering around.

Right knee issues are often linked to resentment and the gallbladder, while left knee issues are often linked to strained adrenals (tiring yourself out, draining your energy reserves).

As we already discussed, the legs and feet are connected to kidney energy; so again, fear is something to consider.

*Tip:* Refer to the root (first) chakra for more.

Liver—Your liver is a big supporter of your immune system. It detoxifies the blood and is also related to hormones and the menstrual cycle. Emotions linked to the liver include anger, resentment, irritability, depression, and frustration, as well as feeling like nothing ever goes right, that your life is a struggle, and everyone is out to get you. The liver is energetically connected to hormones and can affect the endocrine system (specifically women's menstrual cycles) when imbalanced. Liver imbalance can also create pain between the shoulder blades and in the right shoulder. Additionally, stagnant liver energy can create headaches and dizziness, stemming from going over old hurts that we're still angry about.

*Tip:* Refer to the solar plexus (third) chakra for more.

Neck—Emotional energy showing up in the neck can symbolize being frozen in fear, being afraid to turn in any direction, being afraid of making a mistake and heading the wrong way in life, being narrow-minded, having a "pain in the neck" in your life (usually a person), and being afraid to stick your neck out in the world. It can also symbolize being inflexible with yourself, others, and new ways of thinking or being indecisive or not sure which way to go. The stomach meridian runs through the neck and is associated with the emotion of worry. Often, problems with the neck are actually more closely related to the stomach than the neck itself, but it is wise to work from both angles.

*Tip:* Refer to the throat (fifth) chakra for more.

Pancreas—The pancreas secretes insulin in the body. Feelings of bitterness often show up as imbalances in the pancreas. You may also feel like the "sweetness" of life has been taken from you or life has been unfair to you. This can include feeling out of control or victimized. The pancreas can also be affected by the emotion of shock. Pancreatic imbalances might affect the left shoulder and the wrists. Because the pancreas is part of the digestive system, it is wise to think about what in your past is too painful to digest and forgive.

*Tip:* Refer to the solar plexus (third) chakra for more.

**Pineal Gland**—This small endocrine gland produces a number of chemicals and hormones, most notably melatonin. Melatonin modulates the body's circadian rhythm, which regulates sleep. The pineal gland can be connected to sleep disturbances. It is also linked to being unable to balance the cycle of light and dark, metaphorically. This may show up as moods being very high or low, with no balance or rhythm in between.

The pineal gland is also called the third eye because of its connection to psychic sensitivity, intuition, and spiritual dimensions. Refusal to open up to our intuition can affect the pineal gland. Fears around the unknown and what's out there can also affect the pineal gland negatively. These imbalances often show up as migraines, specifically those involving the eyes.

*Tip:* Refer to the crown (seventh) chakra for more. Note: This can be confusing, as the pineal gland is referred to as the third eye but it not part of the third eye chakra.

**Pituitary Gland**—This gland, located at the base of the brain, regulates hormone production in the endocrine system. It is like the control center of other glands such as the thyroid, ovaries, testicles, and adrenals. The pituitary gland is responsible for activating adolescence and the beginning of sexuality, so many times, experiences and emotions from pre-adolescence and adolescence should be looked at. The pituitary gland produces a hormone to prompt the kidneys to increase water absorption, so this gland can be linked to dehydration.

The pituitary gland is affected by confusion, difficulty making decisions, and constantly changing your mind because of doubt and fear. Part of the pituitary is responsible for regulating emotional thoughts, so it is also impacted by emotional instability.

*Tip:* Refer to the third eye (sixth) chakra for more.

**Reproductive Organs**—The reproductive organs are all about creativity, being comfortable with feeling your feelings, security, and joy.

When we do not allow our childlike selves to be expressed (as in being "too responsible"), this can block energy. Similarly, when we are afraid to express ourselves creatively, whether artistically or otherwise, energy can get stuck in these organs. When we have issues and fears related to parenting or being parented, they often affect the reproductive organs as well. Fear or guilt around creating our lives as we wish will affect these organs. Feelings of insecurity (the opposite of feeling secure in the womb) and an inability to turn inward for comfort will affect this area. Other emotions that affect the reproductive system are humiliation, shame, and worthlessness. Repressed emotions about sexuality or energy from past sexual trauma can also show up here. When the reproductive system is imbalanced, it can affect the hips and lower back. I often find that imbalances in the uterus cause discomfort in the shoulder blades.

*Tip:* Refer to the sacral (second) chakra for more.

**Shoulders**—Shoulders, metaphorically, carry weight. Your body might be talking to you about carrying the weight of others, shouldering a burden, giving or being given the cold shoulder, or trying to shrug something off to please others or avoid conflict. Shoulders can also be linked to feeling pushed around.

The energy of the liver is connected to muscles between the shoulder blades and specifically in the right shoulder. Liver imbalances are linked to anger, frustration, and resentment, so these emotions might be worth examining when looking at shoulder symptoms. As mentioned earlier, I have seen imbalances in the uterus manifest here.

*Tip:* Refer to the heart (fourth) chakra for more.

**Skin**—Your skin acts as a barrier between you and the world. When symptoms show up on the skin, they can be linked to feeling like someone is getting under your skin, feeling unprotected against something or someone, feeling that you are itching or burning to release something, and holding hurts right under the surface. Skin rupturing such as blisters can be bubbling-up agitation.

Rashes are sometimes an indication of a burst of anger/expression that you've been holding on to, or the body having a big or sensitive reaction. Skin issues are often linked to the fight, flight, or freeze reaction (panic). Your skin is linked energetically to your lungs, which are connected to the primary emotions of grief, sadness, and confusion. The energy of congestion can also show up in the skin—feeling congested or stuck with emotion and unable to move it out.

*Tip:* I often interpret skin rashes as feeling unsafe and needing to be defensive or protective, so it might be beneficial to refer to the root (first) chakra for more.

**Spleen**—Your spleen metabolizes energy, thoughts, and emotions and is important to immune function. Your spleen is linked to the concept of nourishment and self-support. Issues with the spleen show up as always seeking outside nourishment and not being able to achieve that internally. The spleen is one of the most important organs in Chinese medicine because it's responsible not only for digestion and metabolism but also for the distribution of energy to other areas of the body. The spleen meridian is closely linked to the triple warmer meridian and the fight, flight, or freeze response. When the triple warmer meridian is in overdrive, it borrows energy from the spleen's reservoir, creating a situation where the spleen meridian can't do its job. The spleen is very affected by stress, low self-esteem, and an inability to turn inward. Excessive thinking, worrying, and dwelling drain spleen energy. The emotions connected to the spleen are failure, worry, and helplessness. Imbalances here can affect the left shoulder and mid back.

*Tip:* Refer to the solar plexus (third) chakra for more.

**Stomach/Intestines**—Imbalances in the stomach and digestive system are often related to being unable to "digest" an experience, being sick with worry/guilt/fear, feeling disgusted about something, being gutted (really upset), hating someone's guts, having something eating away at you, feeling stuck or unable to let go of the old (constipation), being unable to metabolize or process something (thoughts, emotions, a situation), or having difficulty slowing down your reactions (diarrhea).

Imbalances in the lower digestive system—such as the large intestine (colon)—are linked to difficulty in letting go and often affect the lower back and hips. Because the small intestine's function is to absorb nutrients, imbalances here can represent being unable to receive and absorb (love, nutrients, etc.), and are sometimes linked to feeling undeserving of those things. Imbalances in the small intestine can affect the lower back and knees.

The neck muscles are linked to the stomach. The stomach is associated with the energy of worry, so if you are a worrier, it will often be your neck and/or stomach that delivers that message.

*Tip:* Refer to the sacral (second) and solar plexus (third) chakras for more.

Throat/Thyroid—The throat symbolizes communication, expression, and metabolizing energy. Symptoms that manifest in the throat can be pointing you to energy around choking on words, swallowing emotions (anger, pain, grief), feeling choked by someone else, being unable to swallow the truth, feeling afraid to speak up, or being choked up and unable to express your feelings. The throat and thyroid can also be imbalanced by speaking, giving advice, and feeling the need to express or defend yourself beyond what feels comfortable or healthy for you.

Thyroid conditions, tonsillitis, and other mouth and throat conditions are most often linked to these types of metaphors.

*Tip:* Refer to the throat (fifth) chakra for more.

### Systems of the Body

While there are many systems in the body, the only two that I interpret as a whole are the nervous system and the immune system. These two are so connected to the functioning of the entire body that I tend to focus on them for a trickle-down effect. The rest of the systems (such as digestive, muscular, lymphatic, and more) are best interpreted by looking at where in the system or in what part of the body, organ, or chakra the dysfunction is manifesting.

**Immune System**—This system is in charge of keeping you safe—keeping foreign invaders out. Symptoms that show up in the immune system are often linked to defensiveness and protection. Do you feel angry and defensive? Do you feel vulnerable and defenseless? What or whom do you feel like you need protection against? (Others, or maybe even yourself?) Or do you feel like you have no protection at all? The immune system is your protector. If you feel unsafe being vulnerable, have no way to protect yourself, or feel defensive all the time, it can wreak havoc on this system.

**Nervous System**—The nervous system is probably the system I focus most of my attention on with clients because its health is so essential to helping them heal. The nervous system is most affected by feeling nervous or anxious about something, being suspended in the fight, flight, or freeze response, waiting for the other shoe to drop, and feeling on the brink of something bad happening all the time. This is related to the triple warmer meridian, which governs the fight, flight, or freeze response. The health of the nervous system is vital to our overall well-being. The nervous system is connected energetically to the bladder, and the bladder is symbolic of being nervous (as in a "nervous bladder"). Because being pissed off is another message the bladder sometimes sends, it's worth looking at feeling nervous about making others upset, which may affect the nervous system. Being too hard on yourself can wreak havoc on the nervous system by creating a situation in which you can never relax (imagine that someone is picking on you all the time—and it's you!). Twitching, spasms, tingling, and stabbing pain that seems to come out of the blue are all messages about energy affecting the nervous system.

### Health Conditions

**Allergies, Sensitivities, and Intolerances**—Allergies are all about feeling fearful and defensive. The body is misdirecting its fear by trying to protect you from things like food and substances that are perfectly safe. This is often a whole-body fear response but can also be connected to strong emotions you were feeling when exposed to particular substances, which then made the body "blame" those substances for the upset and caused an allergy to protect you from them. Working on fear and learning to feel safe will be your biggest assets when working with allergies.

*Tip:* See chapter 10.

**Autoimmune Conditions**—Autoimmune conditions are all about attacking your own body or self. These conditions are often signs of self-criticism, attacking yourself or your past (regrets), and feeling completely out of control. They can be particularly affected by patterns of carrying guilt or shame and feeling unworthy or undeserving.

**Fatigue-Related Conditions**—Fatigue is symbolic of feeling drained and not having "enough" for yourself. It can be linked to feeling tired of life or of a specific situation, being without passion, holding heaviness or sadness, feeling exhausted from never saying no, people-pleasing, and being overwhelmed and drained from cycles of worry and fear. Energy around despair, feeling lost, being stuck with no way out, and overwhelm are commonly seen with fatigue-related conditions. The adrenal glands and their connected patterns are particularly relevant to fatigue.

**Immunodeficiency Conditions**—An underactive immune system can be interpreted as feeling attacked by others or the outside world and not having any self-protection; not being able to defend oneself.

**Inflammatory Conditions**—While pretty much all conditions have a component of inflammation to them, conditions that are specifically inflammatory in nature include arthritis, irritable bowel syndrome, skin issues, allergies, diabetes, heart disease, and cancer. These can manifest as being angry or inflamed, letting old hurts build heat, feeling agitated, being critical toward the self or others, being hypersensitive, or having a sense of impending doom.

**Pain-Related Conditions**—These types of manifestations are often linked to self-punishing patterns such as blaming yourself, feeling like you deserve punishment for not being perfect, holding guilt about the past, absorbing the pain of others, or being hypersensitive about being hurt by others.

**Sleep-Related Conditions**—Insomnia, disrupted sleep, and trouble falling asleep are all related to having an unsettled heart. What is hurting your heart? What is not allowing your heart to feel at peace? Any internal unresolved conflict will affect your heart and ability to rest peacefully.

### Questions to Uncover Clues, Messages, and Metaphors

There are so many metaphors your body could be acting out that will be wonderful clues for your journey. For each symptom or body part, there might be several different messages. Again, my interpretations are just examples and a place to start. It's important to simply start thinking in terms of the body's language and really look at what yours might be saying in the context of your own life. This practice will be invaluable for you moving forward.

Here is a list of questions to ask yourself, which will give you a really good start at figuring out what your body is trying to communicate to you. Make notes of your answers and ideas so you can reference them during your deep clearing work in the next part of this book.

- What is this symptom helping me avoid? If the symptom is in a specific body part, does that part represent something to me that I'm afraid of?

- Is this symptom or condition linked to a fear that makes sense according to the body part or chakra it's located in?

- What does this symptom represent/symbolize that I may be resisting?

- What is the physical function of this body part? Am I allowing myself to do the emotional equivalent of that? Do I fear the emotional equivalent of that?

- How do I feel *about* this symptom or this part of the body? Does that emotion correlate with what could be at the root of symptoms related to it?
- What experience in my past could still be stored in that specific part of my body? Can I use what that part of the body represents in order to figure it out?

You now understand the language of the body and have knowledge that will help you big time in part three, coming up next. The clues you discovered in this chapter will give you a clear lens to help you discover which specific types of stress reactions, themes, and experiences will be most beneficial for you to clear.

*Part Three*

\* \* \* \* \* \* \* \* \* \* \* \* \* \* \*

# Change Your Relationship
# with Stress

Remember how we've talked so much about cleaning up the soil so that big, beautiful tree (you!) can reach an optimal state of well-being? Well, this is how we do it. We change your relationship with stress.

This requires focus on these four main areas:

- Unprocessed experiences
- Harmful beliefs
- Unhealthy emotional patterns
- Fear

For each of these areas, you'll be learning primary techniques to address them:

- Thymus Test and Tap
- Emotional Freedom Technique (EFT)
- The Sweep
- Chakra Tapping
- 3 Hearts Method

You are about to be guided through each of these main areas and techniques in great detail. As mentioned in the introduction, I suggest that you read through and practice them in order to understand them thoroughly. Once you understand the larger picture, you'll be able to determine exactly what works best for you.

The tree analogy we've talked about is the basis of my entire process. We're going to be cleaning up that soil. In chapter 11, I'll be offering you a Healing Tree illustration, along with directions on how to use it, which will help you streamline the entire process. This will be a snapshot of all that you learned in part three.

Let's go!

*Chapter Seven*

\* \* \* \* \* \* \* \* \* \* \* \* \* \*

# Clear Unprocessed Experiences

*You may do this, I tell you, it is permitted.*
*Begin again the story of your life.*
—JANE HIRSHFIELD, *THE LIVES OF THE HEART*

Emotions help us understand our experience, feel alive, relate to others, and so much more. But the trouble comes when our emotions become stuck, the experience of prolonged feelings. When this happens, we feel our emotions intensely, often permanently, without having a way to deal with them—and they create stress reactions.

In this chapter, we'll be exploring the untapped potential of clearing old experiences from our bodies. You'll learn exactly how old feelings remain in our bodies long after we experience them, what their impact is on our well-being, and how to clear them out in order to allow the body to relax and heal. You'll also learn two very powerful techniques for clearing: Thymus Test and Tap and Emotional Freedom Technique (EFT).

## We Are Meant to Let Go of Old Emotions

In my workshops, I put a pen and piece of paper at every seat. I then ask the participants to simply write their name on the paper in front of them. I give them a few seconds and wait until everyone is done. When I look around the room, about half of them are usually still holding their pen in hand even though the purpose of the pen has been fulfilled. This is a great opportunity to explain how emotions work similarly to this task. We are meant to call upon and use our feelings for a specific reason—to express ourselves, to protect ourselves, and more—but once we don't need them for that purpose, we are meant to let them go.

Feelings from our past often remain in the body after their original purpose has been fulfilled. When an animal in the wilderness experiences a stressful event, it shakes, trembles, runs, or does other physical activities to discharge the effect of the stress chemicals in its body. The animal brings itself out of that fight, flight, or freeze pattern by discharging it. It rebalances itself and is then able to go back into nature. The natural human tendency is to do this too, but we are often told (by ourselves or others) to "calm down," "get it together," "stop being so sensitive," "grow up," and "suck it up."

Purging the survival chemicals after a stressful experience sends a message to our primitive brain that we survived and are safe now. This sends a signal to the cognitive brain to process the information and release any associations related to it that are no longer needed. If the energy of facing and surviving a stressful experience is discharged in a healthy way, it can actually help us feel more empowered and able to handle things in the future. It can even help create a sense of security.

If we don't discharge this energy (that is, process and release it), then the primitive brain freezes the experience in our systems. All of the emotions we were feeling at the time remain alive and vibrating inside of us. Candace B. Pert, PhD, author of *Molecules of Emotion*, was the person who opened my eyes to this concept. Her work is based on important findings about how feelings and unexpressed emotions from experiences can get stuck in the body at the level of cellular memory. In *Molecules of Emotion*, Dr. Pert writes: "A feeling sparked in our mind—or body—will translate as a peptide being released somewhere. [Organs, tissues, skin, muscle, and endocrine glands], they all have peptide receptors on them and can access and store emotional information. This means the emotional memory is stored in many places in the body, not just or even primarily in the brain. You can access emotional memory anywhere in the peptide/receptor network in any number of ways. I think unexpressed emotions are literally lodged in the body. The real true emotions that need to be expressed are in the body, trying to move up and be expressed and thereby integrated, made whole, and healed."[10]

## Defining the Unprocessed Experience

The way most of us see and understand "trauma" is only half the story. What often comes to mind when we hear the word *trauma* is abuse, neglect, and catastrophe. But what trauma actually means is a "deeply distressing or disturbing experience." The kind of events we normally consider traumatic are not always the kind of events that actually traumatize us. A traumatizing experience could be something obvious, like a sudden death in the family, or something seemingly less traumatizing, like a hurtful thing your friend said to you on the playground in second grade.

When unprocessed emotions from those experiences live in your body, you may feel them at some level all the time. But here's something else that happens. We also make meanings from our experiences that are not necessarily accurate. These meanings or interpretations then become harmful beliefs that we live by, which you'll be learning about in the next chapter. The unprocessed experience is the reference point or "proof" for the subconscious mind that the belief is still valid for you. You need to clear and neutralize the energies still stuck in your system in order to prove to the subconscious mind that you're okay now and it's safe to relax and move on. This is not necessary for every belief, but for many it will be. Regardless, clearing unprocessed experiences is always beneficial for your well-being.

Let's learn more about what *unprocessed* means. Any disturbing or distressing event or emotional experience in your life that you have not properly *acknowledged, processed,* and *released* may be traumatizing you. This means the feelings from that event are still stuck in your body, or "unexpressed," as Candace Pert refers to them. Trauma, in other words, is less about the event itself and more about it being *unprocessed* and still in your body. So from now on, we're ditching

---

10. Candace B. Pert, PhD, *Molecules of Emotion*, New York: Simon & Schuster, 1999, http://candacepert.com/where-do-you-store-your-emotions.

the stressful word *trauma* and just calling it *unprocessed*. Isn't that less intimidating already?

We can break down what this means even further by looking at the three steps to healing an unprocessed experience: acknowledge, process, and release.

- Any event that you have not **acknowledged** means you most likely said to yourself in some way, even if subconsciously, "Oh, that was no big deal!" when you really were feeling, "Whoa, I'm scared to death" or "That was mighty upsetting!"

- Any event that you have not **processed** means that you don't yet understand it or have not yet come to peace with not understanding it—and it remains unfinished with your spirit.

- Any event that you have not **released** means, because you have not acknowledged and processed it, it might still be stored in your body. If this is true for you, you will most likely feel a "charge" when you recall it. This could show up as a pit in your stomach, a fluttering in your chest, tears welling up in your eyes, a racing heart, sweaty palms, and so on. It is also possible, and even probable, that these events or unprocessed experiences are not ones that you even remember.

Here's my analogy to demonstrate how unprocessed experiences work. Imagine there is a little glass capsule in your body. When you have a stressful experience and don't acknowledge, process, and release it, all of the emotional energy vibrations (feelings), images, scents, and other details get stored in that capsule and remain there. When any current experience or its details match what's inside that capsule, that unprocessed experience can get triggered, "waking it up" in your body. That's when you feel retraumatized, anxious, or a variety of other things as if you were having the original experience again. To take you out of that pattern, you need to find the various triggers and simply clear or neutralize them.

The goal is to get you to a point of accepting that the experience happened, without an intense emotional charge or energy disturbance that accompanies it. You will never have to like or be happy that this experience happened, but you do have to accept it and be at peace with it in order to move on. This goes back to Candace Pert's view that emotions must be expressed and integrated in order to be healed. This will not only help you release that stressful reaction in your body but also allow you to go on to collapse harmful beliefs that were built on the experience.

The really interesting thing is that you may have many of these experiences that you don't even remember, which has caused a bigger challenge for you. These can be things that happened at a very young age, or things that might seem so small you just don't recall them. I'll be showing you how to clear even things that you don't remember shortly.

### Make a List of Memories

A very useful exercise that you can do right now is to make a list for yourself. Jot down all of the experiences in your life that are still bothering you, that you still think of from time to time, or that you wish never happened. What do you remember that you were "never the same" after? What experiences can you recall that you had right before this challenge showed up in your life? What still turns your stomach or makes your heart race when you think about it?

This list may be very long, but it's worth the time to make. This way, you will be able to have a running log and slowly and surely work through it. Do not judge anything as "too small" to go on the list. List everything you can think of. They are all important. I tell clients that I see more "trauma" come from experiences like being humiliated in front of the first grade class than from major car accidents or seemingly more traumatic events. That's because when things are "big," we tend to talk about them, work with them, and process them rather than ignore them.

Your list does not have to be in any particular order or include great detail. Only you need to be able to know what experience you are referring to.

Whether you consider memories from your past meaningful or not, they can be having a big impact on your well-being. It's the same whether you remember them or not. They are always important to clear. And that's probably easier to do than you think.

## Identify Your Unprocessed Experiences with Three Methods

So how do we figure out what's really unprocessed in our bodies in order to release them and move on? You now have a list of memories you made to give you a start. Still, you will need to narrow them down and decide what to work with. There are a couple of solid ways to find experiences that are affecting you most: muscle testing and using your list of memories. Choose whatever works for you; there is no wrong way to go about this.

### Method 1: Muscle Testing

This is my absolute go-to because it requires the least amount of work and is the most accurate. You don't have to remember the experience or need the ability to remain objective in deciding what experiences are really causing an issue for you. You just ask your subconscious mind, which already knows the answers and is just waiting to share the information with you.

With muscle testing, you can use the Standing Test or the Arm Test that you learned in chapter 5. Simply ask your body, "Do I have an unprocessed experience contributing to _____?" You can fill in the blank with "stress in my body." You can also fill it in with the specific challenge you're working with, like "insecurity in social situations" or "difficulty digesting food."

The answer to this question will most likely be "yes." You will probably have lots of these types of experiences, but it only takes one to get the ball rolling. You can then determine through muscle testing at what age this event occurred, getting a clue as to what it could be.

Ask, "Did this event occur between the ages of 0–20? 20–30?" and so on. Keep asking until your body answers "yes" to a specific timeline, then ask about each year within that timeline to get the exact one. Remember to ask the questions slowly and allow your body a few seconds in between to recalibrate.

When you've determined the age, simply stay open and allow ideas to come to you. Remember, it can be anything from an obvious experience, like a death in the family, to something you might consider minor. Just go with whatever comes up.

If you are unsure, you can ask more questions, such as asking what this experience was related to—a person, your career, health, and more. It's really a big guessing game!

Your body will keep answering you, and eventually you will probably remember the experience, or simply have enough information to work with. Even just knowing, for example, that there is an experience from age five that had something to do with school and your teacher will be enough if you can't remember more.

Once you do, it's wise to double-check it through muscle testing. Remember, your conscious mind often thinks it knows what's linked to what, but the subconscious has the final word (and original record). Ask, "Is the experience _____ (describe the experience briefly) contributing to stress in my body?" You can also use anything relevant to you for the last part of this sentence, like "contributing to these migraines" or "contributing to this fear of heights."

Once you get your confirmation, you will have a tangible experience to work with. If you can't identify or recall the specific experience, just identify as much information as you can. Perhaps, through muscle testing, you will end up with information such as having an experience at age twenty that was linked to Mom, but you can't quite figure out exactly what it was about. No problem. Usually the body will allow us to work with just a few key details if we approach it the right way.

> *Tip:* Remember those past-life and generational energies we talked about earlier? Working with unprocessed experiences is one of the opportunities you will have to address those energies. For unprocessed past-life experiences, simply ask your body using muscle testing, "Do I have a past-life experience causing stress in my body?" If you get a "yes," you can use the same process

that you did for getting more information about unprocessed experiences from this lifetime. This just means that the energy of the experience was carried with you from a past life into this one. Just guess what it might be connected to. For generational experiences, ask, "Do I have an unprocessed generational experience that is causing stress in my body?" We are just asking if an experience (and its energy) from one of your relatives was passed on to you. If you get a "yes," you can ask your body which side of your ancestry it came from—your mother's or your father's. Think back to things you know your ancestors went through and see if you can locate the person from whom it was passed, and the experience. To clear past-life and generational experiences, you'll use the same techniques you're about to use for your own experiences, but you'll tweak the wording to fit. I'll explain this more in the coming pages.

### Method 2: Use Your List of Memories

I have two tricks that will help you identify a great experience to work with.

**Determine How You Feel About Your Challenge**—Ask yourself, "How do I feel *about* the challenge I've been dealing with?" The challenge usually refers to the overall issue, such as an illness or panic attacks. This question will help you uncover what unprocessed experiences might be stored in your body and are contributing to your challenge. Do you feel sad? Do you feel frustrated? Do you feel angry? Try to identify just one main emotion that comes up right now. Once you've done that, look at your list. What in your life did you feel this particular emotion about? Perhaps it was a fight you had with a family member or the way something was being handled at work. While there may be several unprocessed experiences, going through this process several times will help you come up with a variety of experiences to work with.

It doesn't matter what type of challenge it is. I consistently find that how we feel *about* the challenge is a good indicator of what kind of emotional contributors helped create it in the first place. An interesting note to add is that when we start feeling better *about* the challenge, this is a great sign of healing.

Here's an example of how this dynamic can play out. Jim came to me with pain in his joints. I asked Jim when this started, and he told me it was about two years earlier. I asked him if he remembered what was going on in his life two years ago. He rattled off a list of things that could have caused his body to go into overload. Once we explored some initial possibilities, I also asked him how he felt *about* the joint pain.

Each person will have a unique feeling about his or her problem, even if the actual problem is a common one, such as joint pain. With Jim, I knew that whatever his primary emotion about his joint pain was would be a good starting point for finding the contributing unprocessed experience.

Jim expressed being "tired of dealing with it." I then helped him figure out what else he was "tired of" or what situation was "tiring" him out around the same time and leading up to that time period (in the previous year or two). You don't need to stick to the two-year time period, but this is just what I did with Jim. We discovered some marital issues around the time that were making him feel "unworthy." With that, we went to work on clearing energy around specific experiences in his past using the methods I'm going to teach you shortly. That helped immensely not only with Jim's frustration and fatigue with the situation but also, in time, with his joint pain.

Over and over again, I find that how we feel physically or how we feel emotionally are very good indicators of the original energy or experience that contributed to the challenge or problem.

**Identify Memories with the Strongest "Charge"**—Here, you can use your list of memories again. What experiences still have the biggest emotional charge for you? Which memories still give you a knot in your stomach or a lump in your throat when you think about them? That's an energy imbalance you are feeling—proof that the emotions or memories are still making a cozy home in your body. Choose the strongest or oldest memories on your list to work with first.

Make sure you allow whatever comes up to just *be*. If you've had significant traumas in your life but one of the things that has the biggest charge is when you didn't win the spelling bee in fourth grade, go with it. The little things can be big, and the big things can be little.

Let me share a story that will help you understand. Sandy, a client of mine, had a really humiliating experience at her first real job after college. She was presenting at a meeting as head of marketing, and started to panic. She didn't typically have to speak to large crowds, especially to the bigwigs of the company. She felt herself start to get dizzy and nauseous, and her palms were sweating. When she made an appointment with me, she was totally panicked, as she had another presentation coming up in a few weeks. I asked her if she'd ever had an issue with public speaking before this, and she said she hadn't really had the opportunity. When I started helping her think on a smaller scale, though, she remembered being extremely nervous several times when she had to stand up in front of the class during her school years. She could consciously recall about five different times, so I asked her to just remember the first one. I knew that the first one would have many others "tied" to it, because all of the subsequent times would most likely be triggering that first experience.

We cleared that first experience, including all of the old feelings, and we didn't even have to touch any of the others. While this won't always be true and you'll have to go back to other experiences you identify, you will sometimes get lucky. For Sandy, all the similar unprocessed experiences that reminded her of the first one came unraveled and released along with it. We must have touched on the "strongest" incident, and when we collapsed that energy, we diffused the rest, too. You'll see how to do this for yourself shortly.

This is a great example of why it's so very important to process and release experiences and emotions from our bodies. If we don't, our current lives become full of trigger opportunities that cause stress on our bodies and often reinforce the beliefs we have from those unprocessed experiences.

Now, we're ready to clear.

## How to Clear Unprocessed Experiences Using Two Techniques

Hopefully you've been able to identify one or two specific unprocessed experiences by now. If you're like I was, you probably have many more than just a few! Let's get started on clearing them. We'll be using two techniques for this, which include Thymus Test and Tap and Emotional Freedom Technique.

I can hear you already... "How will I ever clear all that's happened in my life?" I'm going to sound like a broken record, but I need this to be loud and clear: You don't have to release them all, or all at once. The idea behind this work is to gently (and slowly) release things from your past as they become obvious to you. You don't need to go in any specific or chronological order when clearing experiences. Just like earlier, you can trust that whatever comes up first will be just fine.

I'll teach you two different techniques to clear unprocessed experiences. I use them together in my work with myself and with clients. They are very different techniques, working in different ways. This helps us clean up the experience completely. The combination of them is most effective, at least at first, but after you learn and use them both consistently, you may find that you are able to sometimes clear completely using just one.

### Thymus Test and Tap

The thymus gland, as you first learned in chapter 4, is the master gland of the body's immune system. The thymus gland is located in the emotional energy center of the body, right around the heart, and is the first organ of the body to be affected by emotional stress. In fact, it's often called the "heart's protector." It's responsible, energetically, for regulating energy flow throughout the entire body. It's affected most by emotions related to not feeling safe, feeling attacked by life or others, and the energy of being unprotected. It makes perfect sense why it would be so important in the role of holding (and releasing) unprocessed experiences, right?

The thymus is so powerful, and connected to the rest of the body's energy system, that almost any block or imbalance throughout that system can be affected by working with it. This makes it the star of our next technique. Think of how people naturally "flutter" their chests when they're upset or nervous, or how gorillas thump their chests if they perceive danger. It is believed that there is a natural tendency to strengthen and balance our energy when we need it most.

You might recall from chapter 4 that Dr. John Diamond, a pioneer in the field of holistic healing, believes the thymus serves as the link between mind and body because of its location in the body. You might also remember that the thymus gland is responsible for making T-cells, which are vital to the health of the immune system, including protection against allergies, autoimmune diseases, and immunodeficiency. I believe this makes the health of this gland essential to achieving complete and permanent healing. Candace Pert's work around unexpressed emotions, and years of exploring several ideas to release them, helped me create and perfect Thymus Test and Tap. This technique's ability to process and release feelings, while also rebalancing the immune system in relationship to them, is built upon the healing capability of the thymus gland.

In order to help clear unprocessed experiences, we'll use a simple three-part process:

1. First, you'll identify feelings from unprocessed experiences that are stuck in your body.

2. Then you'll use a simple thymus-tapping procedure to release these feelings.

3. Lastly, you'll install positive emotions to help support the complete integration and healing process for that experience. I usually install positive emotions at the end of a session instead of immediately following work on an experience. Either is okay as

long as you complete or close out your work by installing positive energy.

Remember the metaphorical glass capsule we discussed earlier in this chapter? This technique will help start to clear out the emotions from that.

Let's discuss how the heck we're going to know what specific stuck feelings we still have. By using a list of emotions, along with muscle testing, you can find out what you need to clear.

Let me give you some examples of how this concept works. Naturopaths sometimes use lists of natural remedies (or the actual remedy), along with muscle testing, to detect what is best for their patients. Homeopathic doctors often use lists of various bacteria and viruses, along with muscle testing, to detect what microbes are affecting patients. Integrative nutritionists often use food frequency lists or vials, along with muscle testing, to discover what their clients are allergic to. By using muscle testing to ask specific questions about the lists or vials, trained practitioners can find out what the body needs in order to come back into balance. In fact, long before I knew anything about emotional healing, I was tested for blocking emotions in this very way, and was given essential oils and homeopathic remedies to help me correct them. This same method is going to help us find emotional energies still stuck in the body from unprocessed experiences. Once identified, we will clear them using Thymus Test and Tap.

This list of emotions that we'll be using for the Thymus Test and Tap technique comes from my study and analysis of common emotions that tend to remain long after an experience is over. I left extra space on my list so that if there is a feeling I am missing that you strongly resonate with, you can add it right to the chart for yourself.

You now have the understanding to start clearing.

**Step 1: Rate the Intensity of Your Experience**—Let's first recall an unprocessed experience you identified earlier in this chapter by using either muscle testing or your list of memories. To begin, simply use the title from your list of memories, or create a succinct title for your experience as an easy way to reference it. This might be something like "The day Dad died" or "When Jimmy teased me." If you identified an experience from a past life or an experience passed down to you (generational), make a title for that.

Close your eyes and think of the experience you are focused on clearing. On a scale of 0–10, give it a rating as far as how intense it feels for you, 10 being the strongest. If you can locate where you "feel" it in your body, also take notice of that. It doesn't matter where you are at this moment; it's just good to have an idea of your starting point so you can gauge your progress as you clear. If you don't feel an emotional charge, that's okay.

**Step 2: Identify the Emotions**—You'll begin using the list shown on the next page, along with one of the three methods that follow, to identify which feelings are stuck in your body. You will be identifying and clearing one feeling at a time.

Note: While the emotion of "anxiety" appears on pretty much every other emotion list I've seen out there, it does not appear on my list. I don't consider anxiety an emotion or true feeling. What we often describe as anxiety is simply other emotion that is being suppressed. Suppression of emotions is what actually causes us to feel anxious, uneasy, or unsettled. It feels like something is trying to come up, or out. Without the option of "anxiety" on the list, your body will choose the true emotion that needs to be released. On a separate note, it's great practice for you to consciously learn to identify emotions that you might describe as anxiety so you can be better in touch with what's at the root of it.

*Method 1: Muscle Testing*—The first and best technique you can use to identify old feelings is your superpower of muscle testing. Remember, your subconscious mind is like a recorder. It knows exactly what old feelings on this list may still be linked to the unprocessed experience you are working with. Simply get into muscle-testing position and ask your body this:

| Thymus Test and Tap Unprocessed Emotions ||
|:---:|:---:|
| *Section 1* | *Section 2* |
| Abandoned | Helpless |
| Fearful | Hopeless |
| Grief-stricken | Heavy |
| Unloved | Impatient |
| Intimidated | Out of control |
| Criticized | Defensive |
| Judged | Frustrated |
| Hated | Panicked |
| Berated | Insecure |
| Worthless | Powerless |
| Attacked | Shocked |
| Betrayed | Failure |
| *Section 3* | *Section 4* |
| Rejected | Vulnerable |
| Angry | Unsupported |
| Guilty | Undeserving |
| Resentful | Ashamed |
| Blamed | Overwhelmed |
| Indecisive | Bullied |
| Disgusted | Lonely |
| Conflicted | Alone |
| Confused | Regretful |
| Nervous | Disappointed |
| Unsafe | Discarded |
| Worried | Excluded |
| Hurt | Desperate |
|  |  |
|  |  |

- "Is there an energy [you can use the word *feeling* or *emotion* instead] on this list stuck in my body from _____ (name or title of the experience)?"

  Note: You can alter the wording to whatever is comfortable for you. It doesn't have to be exactly as I've suggested here. I sometimes say, "Is there an emotion from _____ (name of experience) that my body wants to let go of?"

- "Is it in section 1?" If you get a "no," you'll know it's in one of the other sections and you can ask about each of them until you get a "yes."

- Then read each feeling, one by one, asking your body, "Is it _____?" Do this until you get a "yes."

*Method 2: Run Your Fingers Over the List*—Another way to identify the feelings is to close your eyes, take a deep breath, and very gently run your fingers over the list of emotions. If you do it very, very gently, you will actually feel your fingers "stick" a little over the emotion that your body resonates with and wants to release right now. Your fingers are sensing or picking up on it for you.

*Method 3: Use Your Intuition*—Lastly, you can choose emotions on the list and quietly notice which ones jump out at you. Don't judge the feeling and choose from there, but rather just notice what comes up. This method of identifying is least likely to bring up hidden emotions because it's our natural tendency to choose the ones that we think fit or make sense with that experience. We've already learned that it's not always those emotions that are affecting us negatively.

Allow yourself to remember the experience briefly. This is part of the acknowledgment process, but there is no need to dwell on it. We are just momentarily paying attention to it to help go through the processing that didn't happen originally.

You may be used to analyzing and discussing experiences from the past using other approaches. The mind usually desires some understanding before it can let go. However, the energetic body doesn't work in the same way. It will release without it. A brief acknowledgment of the memory lets us essentially hit "rewind" on the experience to go through the steps that we should have gone through originally in order to release it.

**Step 3: Clear by Tapping the Thymus**—Now that you have identified the feelings that are still stuck in your body, you are ready to tap your thymus to clear or neutralize this emotional energy. You will release one feeling at a time, and then repeat.

It can feel good to say the following as you perform the tapping, but it's not necessary at all: *Releasing this _____ (name of the emotion).*

Simply tap seven times firmly over your thymus gland with the fingertips of one hand. As you do this, hold the intention of clearing that emotion while taking a couple of deep breaths. If you are called to, you can repeat the word *clearing* or *releasing*. Again, the verbal cue is not necessary.

Let me give you a breakdown of how and why this method works. The tapping is sending a force of energy through your thymus gland to clear the emotional energy that might be creating a block or imbalance, wherever it is in your system. You don't need to know where it is. Your intention to release it is also a huge part of the actual clearing. You are acknowledging the feeling while giving your body permission to let it go. At the same time that you are tapping your thymus gland to release the emotion, you are also rebalancing and strengthening that gland, allowing it to recover from the imbalance.

You may find that you yawn, sigh, burp, or make some other involuntarily sign of an energy shift. If you don't, that's okay too. After each clearing, you will want to stop and allow your body a few seconds of time, taking a couple of deep breaths.

A single emotional energy that is cleared can free up a huge amount of energy in your system and help boost your thymus gland in a big way, so don't underestimate the power of each release. You may have three feelings to clear for each experience you are working on, or you may have fifty. It doesn't matter. It may take you five minutes, or you may need to work on it over a few weeks. There is no rush.

If you are using muscle testing, you will be asking this each time: "Is there an energy [you can use the word *feeling* or *emotion* instead) on this list stuck in my body from _____ (name or title of the experience)?" As we discussed earlier, remember to revise the wording to something that feels natural to you.

Continue releasing emotional energies related to this experience. After every five to ten energies that you release, take a little break and check in with yourself while visualizing the experience you are working on. Are you feeling better about it? Is the picture less vibrant? Does the emotional charge in your body feel muted? These are all good signs the energy is moving out.

If you are using muscle testing, when your body is done releasing, you will eventually get a "no" response when you go back to test for more. This means that your body has cleared all the feeling that it can for now and needs some processing time. It may also mean that all the feelings are completely cleared. You can continue with step 4 now.

If you don't use muscle testing, you will be using your intuition to know when to stop. Does it feel like it's time to take a break? When you recall the experience, is the feeling or charge associated with it lessening? This means that you're clearing the block or the imbalance related to it. Use your intuition to determine when it's time to move on to the next step.

Remember, when you complete Thymus Test and Tap, you'll be using Emotional Freedom Technique, so you will still have the opportunity to clear more energy from the experience if it's there.

**Step 4: Identify Positive Energy to Install**—Just as we released old feelings using Thymus Test and Tap, we will use it to install positive feelings, too. Installing positive feelings will enhance the work you are doing by giving your body positive emotions to put in the place of what you've released. I like to think of identifying and installing positive feelings as a way to "complete the process" in the body. While it's obviously important to release negative energy, sometimes we can feel empty or like something is missing when we let go of something we've had for a long time, even if it wasn't something we wanted! Remember, thoughts and words are just energy. Using the list of positive feelings on the following page, you will be identifying and installing them one by one. You can do this either by choosing them consciously or, for more accuracy, by using muscle testing to let your subconscious choose exactly what you need at this moment.

*Tip:* Positive feelings should be installed as part of Thymus Test and Tap, but additionally, you can use this technique on its own as a tool to raise your overall vibration. I always end sessions with clients by installing a few positive emotions with them.

If you are muscle-testing, ask your body this:

- "Is there a positive feeling on this list that would be beneficial for me to install now?" If you get a "yes," go to the next question.
- "Is it in section 1?" If you get a "no," then you'll know it's in one of the other sections and you can ask about each of them.
- Then read off each emotion, one by one, asking your body, "Is it _____?" Do this until you've identified your first emotion by getting a "yes." Note: If any of the emotions on the chart pop out for you, you can ask your body about them first to save time.

| Thymus Test and Tap Positive Emotions | |
|:---:|:---:|
| *Section 1* | *Section 2* |
| Able | Comforted |
| Abundant | Connected |
| Accepting | Content |
| Accepted | Decisive |
| Adaptable | Empowered |
| Appreciated | Encouraged |
| Assertive | Energetic |

| Reassured | Flowing |
|---|---|
| At ease | Forgiven |
| Brave | Free |
| Inspired | Grounded |
| Joyful | Happy |
| Light | Deserving |
| Protected | Loved |
| *Section 3* | *Section 4* |
| Secure | Trusting |
| Soothed | Valued |
| Strong | Willing |
| Supported | Calm |
| Grateful | Centered |
| Important | Confident |
| Included | Healed |
| Independent | Hopeful |
| Acknowledged | Open |
| Relaxed | Optimistic |
| Sturdy | Peaceful |
| Understood | Positive |
| | |
| | |

**Step 5: Install the Positive**—Once you've identified the emotion, simply tap seven times firmly over your thymus gland, in the upper area of your chest. As you do this, focus on the feeling. Breathe deeply as you do this. This will "tap" that vibration into your thymus gland and send a force of the positive energy throughout your system.

Just like when you clear old feelings from the past and may yawn, get the chills, or more, you may feel similar sensations when you install positive feelings. I usually install three positive feelings because that feels intuitively good for me. However, you are free to install however many feel right to you.

*Tip:* Thymus Test and Tap can be used for more general clearings, too. For example, you can ask your body through muscle testing if you can release old emotions linked to a specific person, a time period in your life, a specific job, a relationship, a fear you have, or anything else.

### Emotional Freedom Technique (EFT)

This technique came into my life when I needed it most, and I'm hopeful it's going to be the same for you. I now use it all the time, in many different ways, which I'll share later. But for now, we are going to learn how to use it as another way of clearing unprocessed experiences.

EFT tapping works differently than Thymus Test and Tap because we will be working with the unprocessed experience as a whole instead of individual emotional energies. EFT helps us address many different aspects of that glass capsule we talked about. With this technique, we'll be focusing less on individual feelings and more on the whole enchilada—images, sounds, details of the experience, and other triggering specifics.

While Thymus Test and Tap doesn't involve much mental focus on the experience, Emotional Freedom Technique allows us more opportunity to think about the experience and focus on it in greater depth. This is done very safely and without being retraumatized by the experience. With Emotional Freedom Technique, we are more likely to have conscious realizations, cognitive shifts, and perspective changes about the experience during the process. This technique often resonates with people who desire to understand or feel closure about an experience in order to make peace with it and put it behind them.

This can most certainly happen with Thymus Test and Tap, but as you'll see soon, Emotional Freedom Technique gives us the opportunity to walk ourselves through this process in a slower, more conscious way. This can feel more satisfying for some people.

Because these two approaches are so different, it's really beneficial to use them together. Then you get the best of both worlds!

# What Exactly Is Emotional Freedom Technique (EFT)?

Emotional Freedom Technique (EFT) is a technique that combines the principles of acupuncture (without the needles) and talking about unresolved emotional issues—in order to release them. It's a simple and effective tool based on the meridian system, a system of energy pathways in the body, originating in Chinese medicine thousands of years ago. EFT was founded in the early 1990s by Stanford graduate and engineer Gary Craig. Along the meridians, there are special points commonly used in acupuncture that can be utilized to move energy and remove blockages. Where there is an imbalance, there is a corresponding blockage in the meridian system, which contributes to emotional and physical symptoms. Gently tapping with the fingertips works to release the blockages and restore balance.

Gary Craig states that "the cause of all negative emotion is the disruption in the energy system." [11] This may be difficult to comprehend at first because we've learned so much about memories and traumas causing these emotions. However, what he is essentially saying is that it's not the memory or trauma itself, but what happens to the energy system in relationship to that causes the emotions that end up stuck. That is why two people can have the same experience—for example, seeing a bear on a camping trip—and one may feel perfectly fine after it but the other won't. Some of us have more of a propensity for our energy flow to get disrupted or imbalanced during such experiences. By restoring balance to the body's energy system in relationship to memories and experiences, we are essentially reprogramming our relationship with stress.

In simple terms, this is how I see it working. Imagine your dog, Rufus, totally freaks out every time the mailman comes to the door. Each day, you tell Rufus in your most calming voice that he's okay and safe around Mr. Mailman. Chances are Rufus will look at you like you don't know what you're talking about and continue to bark in fear. But, if you kneel down next to him and pat him, calming him at the

---

11. Gary Craig, "What Is EFT? Theory, Science, and Uses," *Official EFT*, www.emofree.com/eft-tutorial/tapping-basics/what-is-eft.html.

same time he is looking at this scary, mean mailman, you'll be sending a strong signal to his body that he is safe and okay even while facing this trauma (Mr. Mailman and his mean mailbag). You'll change how Rufus feels in relationship to or in the presence of this thing that is usually stressful. You'll ultimately change the pattern of what happens to Rufus in his body when he sees the mailman. His system will reprogram itself to be okay and balanced in the presence of Mr. Mailman. We're basically going to do the same thing for you. We're going to change what happens to you in your energy body when you are triggered by something that causes stress.

I'll take a moment here to ask that you tune in to your intuition each time you work with unprocessed experiences. In the case of very sensitive or triggering memories, I encourage you to work with a professional who is trained in this technique. In my own journey, I was able to clear all but one experience by myself. Our bodies often feel safer in the presence of another person who can ground us, and a professional will have extensive techniques to make sure this is a positive experience for you. I do not want you to be afraid to clear things yourself, of course, but please do use careful judgment. Don't work on any severe trauma alone if your gut is telling you to have professional support.

EFT is one of the most diverse techniques I know. If you fall in love with it, you can find a way to use it in almost every clearing you do for yourself. You can take it anywhere, change it to fit your needs, and never have to be without it.

## The Tapping Points

Even if you're already familiar with Emotional Freedom Technique, follow along with me. I do it a bit differently than many practitioners, so you might just learn something new or fun. This technique has endless possibilities, and while I will cover the building blocks and some extra tips and tricks in this chapter, there is much more you can continue to learn.

The first thing you need to know to use EFT is where you will actually be tapping on your face and body. You don't need to do anything with this yet; I just want you to understand where to tap when we're ready.

Just know that, as much as you want to aim for the points I describe, it's okay if you're slightly off. The tapping creates a percussion effect that vibrates through the associated energy pathway, and does the job of clearing. Even kids learn this technique, so I promise it's very easy! Just take it one step at a time.

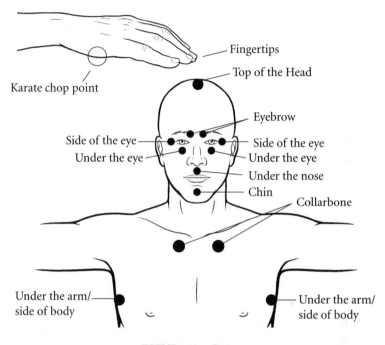

*EFT Tapping Points*

(1) **Karate chop point**—The outside of your hand, about halfway between the bottom of your pinky and your wrist. This is where you would break a board if you were a martial artist.

(2) **Top of the head**—This is smack dab in the middle of the top of your head.

(3) **Eyebrow**—The inside corner of your eye, right where your eyebrow starts.

(4) **Side of the eye**—Outer corner of the eye, right on the bone. It's right inside your temple, closer to your eye.

(5) **Under the eye**—Top of the cheekbone, right under your eye.

(6) **Under the nose**—This is where a moustache would be if you had one.

(7) **Chin**—In the indentation on your chin, halfway between your bottom lip and the tip of your chin.

(8) **Collarbone**—Find where a man would tie a tie, then go out to each side an inch and drop directly under the collarbone.

(9) **Under the arm/side of the body**—This is where a bra band is, about four inches under your armpit on the side of your body.

(10) **Fingertips**—On each finger, tap in the lower right-hand corner of the fingernail, where the nail meets the cuticle. It's not necessary to be precise as long as you aim for the lower right-hand corner.

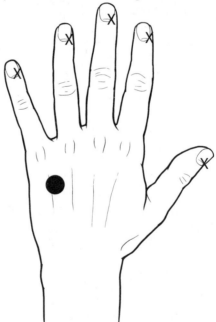

*Top of the Hand (Gamut Point) and Fingertips*

**Top of the hand**—This is often referred to as the *gamut point* in EFT. It's about halfway down the top of the hand in between the pinky and ring finger. Because it's located right along the triple warmer meridian line, it's often used outside of EFT as a tool for neutralizing panic and fear. When you get to this point in your tapping routine, I will be giving you specific instructions on how to use it. For now, you just need to know its location.

For the tapping points that are located on both sides of the body, you can tap on just one side of the body or on both sides. I am a lazy tapper and use only one side of the body. It works just the same, so feel free to do whatever is comfortable for you.

You want to tap about 5–7 times in each spot (just guess; please don't count), and with medium pressure. Feel it out. You can't mess up, so just relax and use this as a practice of undoing your perfectionism. Just make sure you use your fingertips and not your nails. If the points are sore, it generally means the associated meridian is congested and needs to be cleared, so tap gently.

There are various shortcut forms of Emotional Freedom Technique out there, and some skip tapping points to save time. I always use all the points, as each one corresponds with a different energy pathway and different organs, glands, muscles, and more. We want to make sure we cover all the bases and clear all the energy imbalances or blockages related to these feelings. It's not necessary to save ten seconds for a shortcut.

## Tap to Clear Unprocessed Experiences

Now that you have the tapping points down, we're going to go to the next step. Just keep in mind that the ultimate goal of this technique is to (a) bring up the yucky stuff in that glass capsule—sights, sounds, feelings, colors, people, and other details—and then (b) tap to neutralize or clear it in your energy system. That's it. Talk as if you were telling a friend about your experience, and tap. I usually talk out loud, but if you are unable to do this or are uncomfortable with it, you can talk in your head. I think we are all good at that already!

While using Emotional Freedom Technique to clear experiences, being as specific as you can in recalling details will help you get that deep-down-it's-outta-here clearing that we're looking for. If you weren't able to identify the specific experience earlier, hang tight. I'm going to show you how to get a great clearing anyway.

We're going to do this by using a few easy steps:

1. Rate the intensity of your experience.
2. Create a set-up statement.
3. Use your set-up statement while tapping the karate chop point.
4. Tap through the rest of the points.
5. Check in and repeat.
6. Check your work.
7. Wrap up.

### Step 1: Rate the Intensity of Your Experience

Let's start by creating a simple title for your memory or experience as an easy way to reference it. This might be something like "The day I got fired" or "When Johnny told me I was impossible to love." Close your eyes and focus on that memory. Let the feelings come up to the surface (don't worry, we'll clear the uncomfortable feelings along with the unprocessed experience shortly). On a scale of 0–10, give it a rating as far as how intense it feels to you *now*, 10 being the strongest. If you can locate where you "feel" it in your body, also take note of that. Not everyone feels emotion in their body, so if you feel nothing but can just get a sense of or guess your rating, that's all good too. If you are working with a past-life experience or generational experience, you may feel disconnected or unemotional.

It doesn't matter where you are at this moment; it's just good to have an idea of your starting point so you can gauge your progress as you clear.

### Step 2: Create a Set-Up Statement

We always start with what we call a *set-up statement*. There are two parts to this statement, and you will simply fill in the blanks to modify it for your own experience.

*Even though* _____ *(state the experience), I* _____ *(insert a positive idea).*

Using this statement, we are acknowledging the issue we're dealing with but are sending the message that we can let it go, move on, and heal anyway.

**First part of statement:** *Even though* _____ *(state the experience),…*

You want to use as much descriptive detail as possible to "call out" the energy of that experience in your system so it can be cleared. You want to bring it up to acknowledge it so it can be processed and move through your system like it should have originally. It might be something like this:

*Even though Mom forgot me at school after the dance when I was five and I feel this pitter-patter in my heart,…*

If you don't remember your specific experience but have figured out the age at which it occurred or anything related using muscle testing, use a statement such as this:

*Even though something happened to me at age twenty with Mom and I don't remember what it was, I give my subconscious permission to clear it.*

If it's a past-life or generational energy, you could use something like this:

*Even though I have this past-life (or generational) memory of* _____ *(insert details if you have them), I'm willing to release it.*

*Tip:* Try to mix a physical symptom and an emotional feeling into this statement. Think of using this set-up statement as a way to tell the body about the problem you wish to clear.

**Second part of statement:** ..., I _____ *(insert a positive idea).*

Here, you will insert any positive statement to balance the set-up statement. You are essentially telling yourself that even though something bad happened (first part), it is okay (second part).

Here are some examples of positive ideas you can use:

- *I completely love and accept myself.* (This is the most common wording in EFT, but I prefer some of the others, as this one doesn't always seem fitting to the sentence.)
- *I can relax now.*
- *I'm okay anyway.*
- *I choose to release it.*
- *I give my subconscious permission to let it go now.*

Once you have both parts of the statement ready, you can move on to the next step.

### Step 3: Use Your Set-Up Statement While Tapping the Karate Chop Point

To begin the EFT process, you're going to say the entire statement you put together three times in a row as you tap the karate chop point continuously. Use three or four fingers of one hand and tap the karate chop point of the other hand.

You can say the same exact statement three times, or you can vary the wording slightly. As long as whatever you are saying is true for you, it will work.

I always tap with my eyes closed so I can really focus on what's coming up instead of getting distracted by my environment. I try to focus on the old experience or memory in order to help the energy come up to be cleared. However, if your mind wanders, that's okay.

Let's try it now with your eyes closed. Repeat your set-up statement three times. Here's an example:

*Even though Mom forgot me at school after the dance when I was five and I feel this pitter-patter in my heart, I choose to relax now.*

Now you are ready to move on to the rest of the tapping points.

### Step 4: Tap Through the Rest of the Points

Next, you are simply going to tap through the rest of the points you learned earlier while you tell the story of what happened and vent about your experience. By venting, I mean you will pretend you're talking to a friend and just let loose! Talk and talk (while you tap) about whatever is bothering you. Try using a mix of emotional and physical sensations in your descriptions—that is, talk about how you feel emotionally and how it's making you feel physically. It's best to go in chronological order of the story so you can notice what parts of your experience are extra "sticky" for you. As you tap and vent, look at what aspects of the experience are most upsetting. Here's an example.

In an experience where you were bullied, what parts of the story stick in your mind? Perhaps it will be what the bully was wearing, the look on another kid's face when he laughed at you, and the feeling that it would never end. Talk or think about this and tap, focusing on the different segments of your story. It's only when you address all aspects of the story that you'll be able to process and neutralize the experience completely.

It's important to remember that you are simply acknowledging the reality of this experience in order to neutralize or release it. Saying these things out loud will not further embed the experience into your system or make you believe something that isn't already causing an energy disturbance. In fact, tapping will do just the opposite; it will help you release it. Even if I had you tap all day long, saying "I'm scared of kittens," it would never become the truth. And if it is the truth, tapping will help clear it!

Make sure you keep tapping while you recall the details, because even if the experience is painful, you are clearing it. You don't want to sit there thinking about it without doing the tapping (which is probably what you are typically doing even without realizing it). You already cleared at least some of it during the first part of the clearing, when you used Thymus Test and Tap, which should make it less painful to recall.

This round of tapping might include talking about things like this:

- *Concrete details from the experience:* colors, sounds, smells, weather, facial expressions, a certain phrase someone said to you that is upsetting, and so on.
- *Intangible concepts or feelings:* feeling used, being unable to trust yourself or someone else, someone lying, being humiliated, friends ditching you, and so on.

You are just bringing up the yucky energy so it can move out. It may not feel great to temporarily focus on it, but it's the only way to really clear it deeply. Remember, you've been feeling bad about this for a long time as it hangs out in your system, so it's better to deal with it once and for all.

You don't need to use complete sentences. You can use phrases, single words, or descriptions that only you understand. Aim to tap about 5–7 times at each point; or one phrase, sentence, or idea for each point. Just talk about whatever is true and prominent for you. That matters far more than anything else. An example of tapping through the rest of the points might look like the following, but remember to use your own words and feelings.

**Top of the head**—*I can't believe Mom forgot me.*

**Eyebrow**—*I remember being the only one waiting and I was cold.*

**Side of the eye**—*I saw that red van pull up and thought it was her, but it wasn't.*

**Under the eye**—*My friend Amy was laughing because Mom always forgot me.*

**Under the nose**—*I get a pit in my stomach thinking about how scared I was.*

**Chin**—*Mrs. Brown saw me and didn't even try to help. I remember her ugly sweater.*

**Collarbone**—*I am so nervous in my stomach.*

**Under the arm/side of the body**—*Grrrrrrr!* (Noises instead of words are good, too.)

**Fingertips**—*I just wish I had a different mom!*

**Top of the hand**—When you get here, you're going to continue tapping and focusing on the upset while also doing this seemingly silly little routine that helps engage the right and left hemispheres of the brain using eye movements. It's been shown to be extremely useful in releasing and processing old feelings and traumas. Do the following as you continue to tap:

Close your eyes, open your eyes, shift your eyes down and to the right (don't move your head), shift your eyes down and to the left (don't move your head), roll your eyes in a big circle in front of you, then roll them in the other direction, hum a few seconds of a song (anything will do!), count to five quickly out loud (1, 2, 3, 4, 5), then hum for a few more seconds.

Note: I don't do this routine during every tapping round. I throw it in when my intuition tells me to.

Now, repeat tapping through the points from start to finish, just one more time. Just talk out loud, tell your story, and vent about whatever comes to mind again.

Note: If you don't remember the details of your event, you can use the following phrases as you tap the rest of the points and they will work great:

*My subconscious knows exactly what it is.*

*This event at age _____.*

*All the details from that experience.*

*All the smells, sights, and sounds.*

*All subconscious triggers.*

*I know it had something to do with _____.*

*My body remembers the details.*

*Maybe it had something to do with _____.*

What we are doing here is still talking about or guessing about the details of the experience. By suggesting ideas and triggers, the subconscious mind works behind the scenes to find those details and clear them.

If this is a past-life or generational experience, use whatever details you have, such as whom the experience belonged to and more. You can also include the terms *this past-life experience* or *this generational experience* to help fill in the blanks.

You're now ready to gauge your progress in the next step.

### Step 5: Check In and Repeat

Take a break, open your eyes, take a deep breath or two, and check in with yourself. Give the energy a little bit of time to process and shift.

Now close your eyes and tune back in to the experience. Rate your intensity again on a scale of 0–10, 10 being the strongest. Notice if either the physical sensation or the emotional rating has gone down at all. Did it improve? If not, it's no biggie. Occasionally a person will shift with just one round, but most do not. I am my own worst client, as it often takes me many rounds, and then sometimes even lots of processing time after that, to feel a shift in my system. If you aren't feeling any relief, you'll want to repeat the entire process again from the beginning, either with the same words or different words that ring true for you.

If you feel increased intensity after your first round, that's okay. Any change is actually a great sign that the imbalanced energy is mobilizing and transforming. People will often feel a surge in emotion or symptoms as they tap. Again, this is simply because we are bringing things to the surface or stirring them up as part of the release process. They may have been buried deep and are rising close to the surface to be cleared. Hooray! This is exactly what we want.

Do you feel like you're starting to calm down or feel even slightly better about your situation? Sometimes while clearing, release of energy or improved balance will show up in the following ways: feeling less "charge" about the experience, feeling more calm in your body, feeling more optimistic, suddenly seeing things in a way you didn't before, or being more disconnected from the experience when you recall it.

Now repeat the head-to-fingertip tapping and venting for a few more rounds. Take a few deep breaths and focus on the issue again. Rate it and decide if you should keep going. You want to make sure this experience cleared as much as possible, meaning it's no longer affecting you. This will likely require some persistence and repeated tapping, so don't give up.

### Step 6: Check Your Work

It is crucial to check your work. Really test yourself to make sure the experience has been cleared and you're not just shying away from it and wanting to be done. Think of everything that was bothering you before and try to ignite an internal reaction. When you feel neutral or pretty darn close, you can muscle-test to make sure it's clear.

To do this, simply ask your body this question with muscle testing: "Is this _____ (name of experience) _____ causing a stress in my body?"

If you get a "no," the coast is clear. If you get a "yes," simply keep tapping, making sure you cover all of the details, concepts, and feelings that come up for you. Like we talked about earlier, sometimes we need some time to process the work we've done. It's okay to leave this alone and come back to check on it later. It may be easier after a break to assess if there's more work to do.

It's all up to you. You can't go wrong.

*Step 7: Wrap Up*

When you're sure you've cleared your experience completely, or you need to take a tapping break until another session, it's nice to wrap up with some positive tapping. Do not do this, though, until the very end of your session. Tapping and saying positive things all day will not clear anything negative from your system. You need to address things in the way I've described in order to do that.

To close with a positive round, simply do one last tapping round focusing on some positive or calming phrases. It might look something like this:

**Top of the head**—*I am okay.*

**Eyebrow**—*I can get past this.*

**Side of the eye**—*I want to feel better.*

**Under the eye**—*I am feeling calmer now.*

**Under the nose**—*I rock!*

**Chin**—*I'm okay.*

**Collarbone**—*I'm okay.*

**Under the arm/side of the body**—*I'm okay.*

**Fingertips**—*I'm okay.*

**Top of the hand**—*I'm okay.*

That's it!

## How Long Should It Take to Clear an Unprocessed Experience?

You should keep tapping until you feel complete relief. I always joke that even though the intensity scale is 0–10, if you can get down to a 1 that will do it! Many people make the mistake of tapping for only a couple minutes and then say, "Tapping doesn't work." While tapping can feel like a miracle once you learn and use it successfully, it does often take more than a few minutes to get there. Gary Craig says that the three most important aspects of EFT are persistence, persistence, and persistence! You simply need to keep tapping and working through the process as many times as it takes.

When the energy of the experience is truly clear from your system, you will likely have a more distant or faded vision of your memory. It will feel like it happened to someone else or like it's just "there now" instead of holding a strong emotional charge like it did before. However, doing step 6 and using muscle testing to check your work is a great way to be sure.

## EFT Tips

Emotional Freedom Technique really is a wonderful technique, and it's easily adaptable. Here are some points to keep in mind as you practice using it:

- Remember that you don't have to talk out loud when using EFT. This is often helpful, but you can talk quietly in your head if necessary.

- If tapping agitates you for any reason or it hurts your points, use an alternate technique of "touch and breathe." This means, for each point, you'll touch it and take a breath, then move on to the next point.

- Remember that in order to clear the emotional energy, you must bring it up. Don't distract yourself from feeling discomfort during this process.

- Don't jump into positive tapping until you're all finished. The positive round is used only when you're ready to wrap up your session so you can end on a positive note.

- If you don't feel like the old energy is clearing from your system, ask yourself this question about whatever issue you're working on: "Does this remind me of an experience from earlier in my life?" If it does, it's likely that the energy of that experience needs to be cleared in order for you to see improvement in the challenge you're working on. Simply use EFT on that earlier experience in your life. To do this, you'd create and use a set-up statement and then move through the rest of the points while venting about the details of that experience.

I encourage you to keep practicing and reaching new levels of clearing with your work.

## Additional Ways to Use EFT

Now you understand how to use EFT to clear unprocessed experiences. However, tapping can be used for just about anything! I use tapping almost every day for one thing or another. You can use tapping for anything from physical and emotional symptoms to releasing panic and strong emotion in the moment.

While Emotional Freedom Technique is an exceptional technique, clients often get stuck on "what to say" while tapping and are discouraged from using it. While the words you use are not nearly as important as everyone thinks—because bringing up the feeling or emotion is how we actually get effective clearing—this is still a very real stumbling block for some. Here are some alternatives for you to try.

### Use It "in the Moment"

You may often find yourself, in the moment, fearful or upset about something, without the time or ability to do a full clearing session. For these times, a simpler version of Emotional Freedom Technique can be very beneficial. There is no reason you should sit around and feel bad and not be clearing the energy at the same time.

**How-To:** This simple process involves creating and using a set-up statement to verbalize how you are feeling now, then going through the rest of the points while venting about that same thing. You'll use the set-up statement three times while tapping the karate chop point continuously. When you've done that, simply tap through the rest of the EFT points and vent about it. As long as what you're saying is true for you, you're doing it right. Remember to include how you feel both physically and emotionally, if both apply.

If you ever need to use this technique in a place where you're unable to tap on all of the points, simply put your hand in an inconspicuous place and tap on the fingertip points only.

### Utilize Reminders from Your Past

Sometimes it's difficult to work on a traumatic event from your past because it's just too scary, you don't recall details, or you are maybe too detached to conjure up the feelings in order to clear them.

**How-To:** Use any other means you can think of to bring up feelings associated with what you want to clear. These might include tapping while reading past journal entries aloud, writing out your story or feelings and then tapping as you read and reread them, recording your experience or feelings with your voice and tapping along to that, and playing songs from your past that evoke emotion so you can tap along to that.

### Ask Your Subconscious Mind for Help

Calling on your subconscious mind for help is a great way to get some deep clearing, even if we don't know exactly what needs to be cleared. Remember, the subconscious mind knows everything.

**How-To:** Recite a short intention or prayer asking that your subconscious mind come to your rescue and help you clear. Something like this will do just fine:

*I trust and allow my subconscious to help me clear this challenge. Thank you!*

An example set-up statement might look like this:

*Even though I have no idea what is holding me back from healing, I give my subconscious permission to release it anyway.*

For the rest of the tapping points, focus on whatever issue you are clearing, trying to incorporate the emotions you feel and any information you have.

Tapping through these points might look something like this:

*"I don't know what's making me anxious." "Maybe it's _____ (insert any guesses)." "My subconscious knows." "I just can't figure it out."*

Just keep tapping and talking out loud, which will trigger your subconscious into pulling up whatever it needs to help you clear.

### Incorporate Metaphors

As you've learned, symptoms are metaphors or clues from our body. They are our body's language. Using the guide I've given you, and your own intuition, you can work some of these ideas into your tapping.

**How-To:** Incorporate any metaphors or clues that might apply to you from chapter 6 into your set-up statement and tapping.

Here are a couple examples of what a set-up statement might look like:

*Even though I can't digest what happened to me when _____, ...*

*Even though I'm so mad that this grief from _____ is suffocating me, ...*

*Even though Mom stabbed me in the back, ...*

Remember that the more you practice using EFT in various ways, the more comfortable you'll become using it. There's no right or wrong way to do it as long as it's working for you.

In the next chapter, we'll be learning how to release harmful beliefs, which often come from the unprocessed experiences we've just worked with.

## Prevent Unprocessed Experiences in the Future

Now that you understand a lot about unprocessed experiences and how they get stuck in the body, let's talk about how to prevent them in the future.

First and foremost, be conscious of how you're feeling. Really allow yourself the opportunity to feel your feelings and acknowledge your emotions. Don't give in to the temptation to tell yourself, "It's no big deal!" even if you wish it wasn't. Acknowledge how you're feeling and accept it, even if it doesn't make logical sense or you don't like it. In her book *Bird by Bird*, Anne Lamott shared this advice from her therapist:

"She said to go ahead and feel the feelings. I did. They felt like shit." This says it so beautifully because feelings aren't always pleasant; but if we can allow and accept those feelings anyway, there's a much greater chance that they'll feel like shit only temporarily instead of for a lifetime.

You can also use EFT during moments of stress, as we just discussed. This immediately helps your body calm down instead of going into, or staying in, fight, flight, or freeze mode. In addition to EFT, other practices that help our bodies release emotional energy are massage, meditation, hot baths (especially with essential oil), dancing, deep breathing, and exercising.

*Chapter Eight*

\* \* \* \* \* \* \* \* \* \* \* \* \*

# Release Harmful Beliefs

*Science teaches that we must see in order to believe,*
*but we must also believe in order to see.*
—BERNIE S. SIEGEL, *LOVE, MEDICINE & MIRACLES*

Harmful beliefs are where I find the jackpot with most clients. Most of us, and I was no exception, have many reasons *not* to heal. This is because our challenge may actually benefit us in some way, or we believe deep down that it does. I know that might sound a bit ridiculous, but by the end of this chapter you'll understand it very well.

In this chapter, you'll first become familiar with what harmful beliefs are and how they might be showing up in your life. Toward the end of the chapter, I'll teach you two techniques to help you clear those beliefs that are blocking you:

- The Sweep
- Chakra Tapping

While doing the work to uncover these beliefs can be painful, if you add some humor and curiosity to the process, it can actually become entertaining. I consider myself a harmful beliefs detective now, and soon, you will become one too.

## How Beliefs Can Block You

Do you have a pattern of feeling worse the more you try to feel better? Have you tried everything and it feels like nothing is working? Do you begin to improve and then suddenly have a flare-up of your emotional or physical symptoms? Do you struggle with a pattern of self-sabotage, even finding it difficult to help yourself when you know you need to?

If this describes you, I can almost guarantee that *you* are getting in your own way of overcoming whatever your challenge is. I know this may be hard to swallow. Just stick with me and I promise this will be the best truth you ever entertained the possibility of.

Your subconscious mind might be blocking you from not only your treatment efforts but also your healing ability. One reason this happens is because, at some level, you actually have an inner conflict about healing. This type of inner conflict occurs when one part of us wants to change, but the other part (often the subconscious) does not want to change because it believes the change is not good for us. Simply put, it's a resistance to your goal, which sabotages your efforts.

Even though your conscious mind is doing everything it can think of to heal, your subconscious mind may be holding what it thinks are very good reasons *not* to heal or overcome your challenge. Part of you may see the challenge or illness as an upside or benefit, which is better in some way than being well. This means you perceive there is a benefit to your challenge.

Exploring harmful beliefs was the single most important action I took in my own healing journey. It has proven over and over again in client sessions to be essential to the healing process for others, too. In the same way you unsubscribe to emails that don't feel good, create stress in your life, or have views you don't want to be connected with, you can unsubscribe to your own beliefs.

As you learn about harmful beliefs, the most important thing to remember is not to judge yourself for them. We make meanings from the world around us; those interpretations and perceptions are recorded by the subconscious mind and then become the beliefs or rules by which we live—often without us being aware we are doing so. The problem arises when we carry these beliefs into our adulthood.

Many of the beliefs that are blocking you won't make logical sense, at least at first. In fact, some could probably be categorized as shocking. All of this is awesome news, though. As with my own healing, you'll be discovering blocks you never thought of. This will give you the opportunity to work on things you never knew existed, taking new directions and getting results you've never gotten. The big-picture idea here is to slowly release all the subconscious reasons that your body, mind, and spirit have to *not* heal. There will probably be a lot of reasons, and that's okay. We'll get through them, one by one.

Illness or emotional challenges often arise after we've been living in a way that's not true to who we are. This would include being in a relationship we know is not healthy, "dimming our light" or softening our personality for others, or doing a job we feel is unethical or not in line with our true selves. A lot of times we are living in this way because there are harmful beliefs driving our train.

Early childhood experiences are the first way we get ideas or beliefs about life and ourselves. Beliefs are not fact. Beliefs are based solely on our generalizations from the past, experiences, other people's messages about us, and the meaning we make from those experiences. Unfortunately, we don't consciously decide what we believe—which means a lot of B.S. is stuck in those brains of ours.

Let me show you how this works. Let's say you are four years old and you draw something you are very proud of. You arrive at home excited from preschool and show your mom, who is busy trying to finish her own stuff and take care of your baby sister. She smiles and abruptly tells you to go put it away and get ready for dinner. This type of scenario plays out in a few different scenarios that week because your dad is out of town for work and your mom is preoccupied with all her responsibilities. You may feel rejected and perceive not that your mom is simply busy, but that you are a terrible artist. You then start looking for evidence of this as you grow up. Your subconscious mind takes in that new rule you've made: *I am terrible at art.* Then you go through life with that perspective, directing your behavior according to that belief. This experience might translate to you being closed off to your creativity, feeling ashamed to express yourself, and more. Healing is, in part, about unlearning or unbelieving anything that doesn't help you feel good. Your younger self saw things in one way, but now you're older. Unless you would allow a four-year-old to run your life (oh my!), it's probably time to update your mental records.

The subconscious mind is not critical or judgmental; it does not analyze or reason. It simply gathers data and then acts according to the conditioning, programming, instructions, and messages it receives. Thousands of these interpretations of experiences from when we're young become beliefs that then become rules for our lives. Our subconscious mind uses these rules to direct our behavior. As we keep going back to those memories, experiences, and interpretations of the past, we create new cells along those neural pathways reinforcing that old belief and response pattern. These beliefs are one of the largest impediments to healing. The good news is that releasing these beliefs can help create new, healthy patterns.

Harmful beliefs work like this:

- They create a tainted lens through which we start to see our lives and ourselves, skewing our perceptions.
- This lens keeps us stuck in life-limiting thoughts and patterns.
- Believing these limits, we continue to live within the confines of them, further fulfilling that belief, which helps create our reality.
- Beliefs create a pattern of self-sabotage.

Let me give you an example of this phenomenon. Joe was a new client who was also new to energy work. He'd been married to the love of his life for ten years, but had been experiencing some anxiety and severe digestive issues. His wife sounded really fun, and he described her as the "life of the party," often stealing the show in any group setting. This was something he really loved about her, as he tended toward the shy side. However, as Joe and I got talking, he admitted that he became shy after an experience at a school dance when he was young. All the other kids were in groups, and no one invited Joe to join them. He spent the entire dance hanging out around the food table alone, going to the bathroom, and even tying and re-tying his shoes just to look busy.

I have heard various forms of this story from many, many clients, and I think most of us can relate to it. Ever since then, Joe had been uncomfortable in social situations and terrified of being excluded. He felt like it was time to get back to being his true self and not being the "dud" at parties. We worked on releasing the unprocessed experience of the school dance in our first session. This experience could have created a belief such as "I'll be abandoned at parties." I muscle-tested to check a few beliefs, including that one, and we got a "no" for everything I could think of. So then we came up with some other ideas that were not related to that specific dance.

As we brainstormed, we muscle-tested one belief that I see often: "If I am my true self, it will threaten a relationship." Yep, that was it. His body gave us a "yes." So we started muscle-testing for relationships and found out that his body was linking this fear to his wife. Joe told me that this belief actually resonated at a conscious level, too, so even without muscle testing, we may have eventually gotten there. He was actually blocked from moving past this because deep down he believed that if he was his true outgoing self, it would threaten his wife and her big personality. He believed at a subconscious level that they couldn't both be the "fun ones." He told me that he could have perceived this from his own parents' relationship, where his mom was the "talker" and his dad was the one who stood by quietly. When his dad would speak up, his mother would berate him in front of others. Whether this turned out to be an actual issue in his own marriage or not, it was extremely stressful to Joe's body to be suppressing his own personality for the sake of his wife.

Clearing the unprocessed experience of the dance using Thymus Test and Tap and Emotional Freedom Technique was a great start. We then cleared two other experiences he remembered about his mom embarrassing his dad for speaking up and trying to participate in conversations. We chose one by picking the earliest and strongest memory, and the other by using muscle testing to narrow it down. Next, we worked on the belief "If I am my true self, it will threaten my relationship with my wife," using techniques you'll learn shortly. This helped Joe feel much more comfortable in social situations.

Because you now know how to interpret the body's language in relationship to symptoms (from chapter 6), I'll share this interesting side note. The digestive issues Joe was experiencing were very specific to this situation. Although the digestive system is greatly impacted by stress reactions of all kinds, Joe's digestive system was also acting up as a protection mechanism, as it prevented him from going to places where he might have to wait in line for a bathroom. This was very convenient, in a way, as it helped him avoid situations that triggered his social fears. Can you see now how closely unprocessed experiences, harmful beliefs, and physical symptoms are connected? We are just complex puzzles that need to be lovingly solved.

The subconscious mind can have programming that is making us believe that a challenge, symptom, disease, or problem is actually *better* for us than being free from it. Joe's fear in social situations and digestive problems were manifesting in an effort to protect his marriage.

Beliefs can affect us in so many different ways. As you become aware of the beliefs in your own life by observing your experiences that come up, be open-minded and entertain all possibilities. In my work with clients, I often hear, "Really?! It's that?" when we find some of these.

## The Power of Belief

I want you to see just how important it is to spend time on beliefs, as if your life and health depend on it. In fact, they do.

One of the most convincing stories of the power of belief I've heard comes from the story of Sam Londe, who was diagnosed with cancer of the esophagus.[12] In 1974, this type of cancer was considered fatal. A few weeks after his diagnosis, Sam died. When the autopsy was done, it was revealed that Sam had very little cancer in his body, at least not enough to kill him. There were a few spots scattered around his body, but no cancer at all on his esophagus. Dr. Clifton Meador, his physician, stated, "I thought he had cancer. He thought he had cancer. Everyone around him thought he had cancer … had I removed hope in some way?"

---

12. Desonta Holder, "Health: Beware Negative Self-Fulfilling Prophecy," *The Seattle Times*, January 2, 2008, http://seattletimes.com/html/health /2004101546_fearofdying02.html.

In 2014, the *New England Journal of Medicine* published a trial showing that mimicking surgery can be as effective as the real thing.[13] In this study, patients were candidates for knee surgery, with a torn meniscus and debilitating pain. When they arrived in the operating room, study surgeons in Finland performed either a meticulous repair of the torn cartilage or make-believe surgery. Incisions were made, and closed, with no other intervention. In case anesthetized patients could hear or understand, the doctors and nurses passed instruments making the typical sounds you'd expect, and pretended to do surgery for as long as the procedure would normally take. Patients who underwent real surgeries and patients whose surgeries were faked had equal improvement.

In Bruce Lipton's book *The Biology of Belief: Unleashing the Power of Consciousness, Matter, and Miracles,* he tells a story that demonstrates the absolute power of belief. Interior designer Janis Schonfeld took part in a clinical trial to test the efficacy of an anti-depressant drug.[14] The pills relieved her thirty-year experience with depression, and the brain scans confirmed that the activity of the frontal precortex of her brain was greatly enhanced. Only at the end of the trial did Janis find out she had been taking a placebo and not the real drug. Her belief about what the drug would do for her was responsible for her improvement.

There are endless findings now that demonstrate that our beliefs actually create our reality. Dr. Lipton's groundbreaking research is perhaps one of the most awe-inspiring examples, proving that your mind will change the biology of your body according to your subconscious beliefs. Your body's chemistry looks to that dominant part of your brain for direction. Do you see why it's so essential that the beliefs you hold are good for you?

---

13. Raine Sihvonen, MD, et al., "Arthroscopic Partial Meniscectomy versus Sham Surgery for a Degenerative Meniscal Tear," *New England Journal of Medicine* Vol. 369, No. 26 (Dec. 26, 2013): 2515–2524, www.nejm.org/doi /full/10.1056/NEJMoa1305189.

14. Bruce H. Lipton, PhD. *The Biology of Belief: Unleashing the Power of Consciousness, Matter, and Miracles* (Santa Rosa, CA: Mountain of Love/Elite Books, 2005), p. 111.

Clearing harmful beliefs so you can be in total alignment with healing is your newest tool to freedom. Now, are you ready to start?

## Determine What's Behind Your Beliefs

We'll learn to clear harmful beliefs at the end of this chapter, but first we need to figure out what's behind your beliefs. As you work on discovering blocks, I recommend that you keep a notebook to use as your own I-can't-believe-that's-in-my-brain journal. Jotting them down as you think of them will help you start the flow of ideas and also create a list to work from as you clear.

Beliefs that block healing, due to the subconscious not being in alignment with healing, are typically built around some main concepts.

Safety (It's unsafe to heal)—If part of us doesn't feel safe to heal at a core level, it can act as a monster-size block. This is the block I see most often. I know this one seems illogical, as illness or emotional challenge typically makes us feel very unsafe. However, there are definitely ways that we perceive it does keep us safe, too. These types of issues often keep us out of the big, bad world and home in our safe zone, help us say no to things we otherwise might not, and more.

Willingness (I'm unwilling to heal)—This covers the idea that we aren't willing to do what it takes to heal, energy-wise, financially, or otherwise. This block has to do primarily with the "work" involved in healing. This is not a belief based on laziness, but often comes from being drained of gusto after a long dance with our challenge.

Deserving (I'm undeserving of healing)—This block is all about believing that we don't deserve to heal or be happy and that we are not worthy of it. This is often centered on our not feeling good enough.

Readiness (I'm not ready to heal)—Not feeling ready to heal can play a part when we feel like things would change too fast, or there is more we need to do before we are ready to get back to life.

**Ability (I'm unable to heal)**—This block is centered on believing you don't have it in you or don't have what it takes to heal; that you aren't able to heal because you don't have either the internal or the external resources to do so. This block is linked to the thought or belief that "others can heal, but I can't."

**Possibility (It's impossible to heal)**—Feeling like it's not possible to heal is a belief that comes many times from the medical professionals who are trying to help you. Hearing things like you have the "most severe case" of something or that your issue is "incurable" will give ammunition to these types of beliefs. This block is built around feeling like your circumstances are just too bad.

**Wanting (I don't want to heal)**—Not wanting to heal usually results from having an upside to your challenge. Everything that we perceive as negative in our lives (such as illness) also has a positive aspect (a benefit). Sometimes, even if only at a subconscious level, the benefit we gain from the challenge prevents us from wanting to overcome the challenge.

The important thing to know here is that there may be a ton of beliefs to work on. I mean, like mountains of them. Clearing beliefs is a marathon, not a sprint. You can only clear as fast as the beliefs reveal themselves to you. You won't have to conquer every last one in order to heal. You just need to make a good dent in the pile.

## Narrow Down Your Beliefs

Let's say you have an overarching belief that it's "unsafe to heal." You may need to explore lots of sub-beliefs, or whys, to your one overarching belief. In other words, there may be several reasons why your body feels like it's unsafe to heal. Examples include things like "Someone I know will be negatively affected by it," "I will have to find a new job," and "I won't get as much support from Mom and Dad." Do you see how these are all beliefs, but some could also be considered benefits or upsides to your challenge? You're always looking for both.

The following example list will open your eyes to the vast number of possible harmful beliefs that could be making it difficult to heal. Remember, they will likely fall into one of the major categories (safety, willingness, deserving, readiness, ability, possibility, or wanting), but the reasons behind them can be plentiful, and varied. I'm going to start you with a list here so you can brainstorm from it. Also feel free to use each belief as a suggestion and change some of the words to those that would be more fitting for you. Just as I explained when we cleared unprocessed experiences in the last chapter, you don't have to clear or release all of your beliefs to heal. I certainly could still find some hidden ones for myself if I tried. Don't let this process overwhelm you. Just start somewhere.

Here are some examples of beliefs that block healing:

- *I'll only be loved if I'm sick.*
- *I'll only be loved if I'm perfect.*
- *I'm unlovable.*
- *I am undeserving of love.*
- *I don't matter.*
- *I am worthless.*
- *I always make the wrong decision.*
- *When things start to go well, something bad happens.*
- *If I do what I want, other people will be unhappy.*
- *Being healthy and happy at the same time is impossible.*
- *I need this challenge or illness to have my needs met.*
- *I need to be sick to feel safe.*
- *I deserve to be sick/unhappy because of something bad I did in the past.*
- *Being sick/unhappy is my punishment for doing something bad in the past.*
- *If I heal, it will just come back.*

- *I'll end up alone if I heal (people only stick around because they feel bad for me).*
- *It is unsafe to relax.*
- *It is unsafe to be happy.*
- *If I do something good for myself, someone else will be upset.*
- *I'll want to leave my relationship if I heal.*
- *I can only heal with more support.*
- *I'm only worthy when _____ (I'm perfect, I am doing things for others, etc.).*
- *I can only heal with more money.*
- *If I get well and still can't find a partner, I'll have no excuse.*
- *Healing would prove this was my fault in the first place.*
- *I will be too vulnerable if I heal.*
- *I'll have nothing to do anyway if I heal.*
- *There's no point to healing (I have no purpose worth healing for).*
- *I have to forgive others in order to heal and then they'll be off the hook.*
- *I will lose my identity if I heal.*
- *I need this illness or challenge because it makes me special.*
- *I am too far behind to ever catch up if I heal.*
- *I'll have to live up to others' (or my own) expectations if I heal.*
- *I'll have to be perfect to make up for all of this.*
- *I'm going to let myself down.*
- *I might lose my friends if I heal.*
- *I don't know how to heal.*
- *People will take care of me only when I'm sick.*
- *I'll have to be more assertive if I heal.*
- *I'm not strong enough to heal.*
- *I don't have what it takes to heal.*

- *I'm too sensitive to heal.*
- *I'm too delicate to heal.*
- *I'm unable to handle treatments.*
- *I need this challenge or illness as a distraction (from my unhappy life, my marriage, my job, etc.).*
- *It's unfair to the other people who are still suffering if I heal.*
- *My life will change if I heal (and that's too scary).*
- *I'll hurt my doctor's/friends'/family's feelings if I don't heal their way.*
- *I'll have to be successful if I heal.*
- *I'll have to leave an unhealthy relationship if I heal.*
- *It's too much work and I don't have the energy left to heal.*
- *I'll lose my financial benefits if I heal.*
- *I might lose my support system if I heal.*
- *Nothing will work anyway.*
- *People only believe I'm in pain if they see me suffering physically.*
- *I've always had this problem and I always will.*
- *I'm not good enough to heal.*
- *Everyone else is smarter than me so it's easier for them.*
- *I'm too damaged to heal.*
- *Someone has to suffer and maybe it's meant to be me.*
- *I can grow spiritually only when I'm sick/unhappy.*
- *I need this illness or challenge as an escape from family, work, or more.*
- *I need this illness or challenge because it's the only way I can say no.*
- *Getting better will hurt my relationship with someone I love.*
- *My life will be too stressful if I'm healthy.*
- *I'll have to be social if I heal.*
- *I won't have excuses if I fail or quit something.*

- *I will have to live up to my full potential if I heal.*
- *No one will take care of me if I heal.*
- *I will need to figure out my life if I heal.*
- *I will have to be intimate with my spouse if I heal.*
- *I will have to be present for my children if I heal.*

Are you starting to see that nothing is off-limits as far as beliefs go? Good. That's going to help you big time during this process.

## Key Questions to Identify Harmful Beliefs

During client sessions, I have "random" beliefs come to me intuitively all the time. Although they sometimes seem silly or farfetched, they often turn out to be true for my client and really help us move forward.

Now that you have a good solid start, see what comes up for you when you ask yourself the following questions, which are designed to trigger ideas for beliefs. If an idea pops into your mind, go with it—it means something. If an answer comes that seems ridiculous, go with it too—it's your subconscious mind trying to push clues forward to you. When a memory or belief pops up, write it down. We'll learn about clearing them away in the next step.

- Why could part of me believe I *need* this illness/injury/situation/ challenge?
- If I give this up, who won't be punished anymore that I think should be?
- Who would it hurt if I got over this issue?
- Do I feel more powerful in some ways with this problem?
- Does letting go of this mean I am forgetting something, or forgiving someone?
- What would I lose without this "story"? What is the downside?
- What do I think I have to do to make this situation go away? Is there a downside to that?

During my own healing process, I would often ask myself, "If my brain had some crazy idea of why I shouldn't heal, what would it be?" You'd be surprised what answers might come to you.

Another excellent way to identify beliefs is to use your superpower of muscle testing. Simply ask your body the questions I just suggested, and keep asking them until you lead yourself right to the belief. Remember, your body will tell you what's true for you. If you don't think it's beneficial for that to be true, it's something that needs to be released or shifted, which we'll be doing shortly.

Muscle-testing to identify a belief might go something like this:

Ask, "Would I hurt someone if I healed from this _____?"

If your body says "yes," you can continue asking.

Ask, "Would I hurt Dad if I healed?"

If your body says "no," keep guessing with family, friends, colleagues, and whoever else comes to mind.

> *Tip:* This is a place where generational beliefs can show up. If you suspect this, you might want to use muscle testing to check it out. Ask something like, "Is there a generational belief causing stress in my body?" (Remember, you can revise the question to address whatever challenge you are currently working on to be more specific than "stress in my body"). If you get a "yes," you'll have to figure out what it is based on what you know about past generations.

When coming up with beliefs, you'll want to try to use positive statements, like we did with muscle testing, so as not to confuse the body during the clearing process. That means instead of "I won't have my needs met without this illness or challenge," you'd want to work with the belief "I can only have my needs met when I have this illness or challenge." As another example, "I always make the wrong decision" is clearer than "I never make the right decisions." When muscle-testing, using the clearest form of the belief will really help ensure that all of your responses are accurate.

Hopefully you now have a head full of beliefs swirling around. The subconscious mind usually has lots of "great" (or so it thinks!) ideas on why we shouldn't overcome our challenges.

We're going to talk about exactly what to do with these harmful beliefs now.

## Find Out If You Need to Know More

With some beliefs, the only requirement from our body to clear them will be to simply be aware of the beliefs themselves. For other beliefs, our bodies will not let them go until we identify the origin point of each belief—in other words, where the heck it came from in the first place. Because beliefs come from our early experiences, where we gathered most of our data about life, this means we'll need to find the original unprocessed experience each belief was built on.

I have not been able to find a specific reason as to why the body will require us to identify some experiences before it will let go of the beliefs attached, but will not require us to do the same with other experiences. The interesting thing I've seen over and over again is that there is more of a propensity to understand and dissect beliefs when we start this work, but over time, the body becomes more focused on just clearing and letting go. It's as if the subconscious mind says, "I don't need to know every little detail. I trust this process now!"

Either way, it's important to find out what it will take for your body to let go of each belief in order to move forward. There is really only one way to know for sure, and it's through muscle testing.

Here's what to ask using muscle testing: "Do I need to know more about the belief _____ (state the belief) before I can release it?"

If you get a "yes," your body is saying there is more that needs to be brought to your attention before you can really heal from it, and that's okay. I often joke with my clients about this, reassuring them that they simply have a "nosy" subconscious that day. No big deal. Use muscle testing and ask, "Do I need to find an unprocessed experience that created this belief?"

If you get a "yes," what you're going to do is jump back to chapter 7 where you learned how to find and clear unprocessed experiences. Use the process of finding unprocessed experiences but alter the muscle-testing question to refer to the belief you are working with. It might look something like: "Is this belief linked to an experience that happened between the ages of 0–20?" Continue like this until you figure out the age and the experience. You are essentially going back to find where your body got the idea that this belief was true. Then, once you've found and cleared the experience, come right back and you'll have done all you need to continue.

If you get a "no" from your body about needing to work with an unprocessed experience, your body is saying that you need to know something else about the belief. This is often a process of guess and check. Using muscle testing, ask if the belief is linked to a person. Or maybe it's connected to school. Just keep guessing until you get some more details.

When you get a "yes" for one of your questions, repeat this question: "Do I need to know more about the belief _____ (state the belief) before I can release it?"

Eventually you will get a "no," which means your body is ready to release the belief. It has brought to light all that it needs to.

Note: If you are still working on the art of muscle testing and are not confident in it quite yet, you can err on the side of caution and assume your body is saying, "Yes, I'm nosy and I need to know more." Go back to chapter 7 to find and clear unprocessed experiences related to the belief, then come right back here when you're ready to continue. Remember, it will never hurt to clear experiences, so even if it's not absolutely necessary to this process, you can be sure it's benefitting you in some way.

For generational beliefs, it's usually not necessary to find a connected experience, but it can be good to check.

## Clearing Harmful Beliefs with Two Techniques

Like most energetic imbalances, harmful beliefs can create big blocks, but they usually aren't all that difficult to release. Phew. There are just a few parts to successful reprogramming:

- **Acknowledgment.** Are you seeing a pattern here? We need to acknowledge that we have this belief and that it's not working for us anymore. Sometimes we need to acknowledge the origin of this belief—whether it be a specific event in our lives, something someone said to us, or another source.

- **Trust.** Talk to your subconscious mind like a trusted, compassionate, kind companion. We need the subconscious mind to feel safe enough to relax and accept these directions to release old beliefs.

- **Replacement.** Find a new or healthier belief you want to install or replace for the subconscious mind to use instead. We want to offer it another, more fulfilling option instead of leaving it void.

You are going to learn two very effective ways to clear beliefs: *The Sweep* and *Chakra Tapping*. This will give you wonderful options to use. These techniques can be used independently or, if needed, as a powerful combination.

### The Sweep

*The Sweep* is a simple technique that clears beliefs by gently sweeping them right on out of the subconscious mind.

The subconscious and conscious minds are designed to work together, like a buddy system. As you know, the subconscious mind's programming originated in experiences, thoughts, and messages. In other words, it's open to influence from the conscious mind and our perceptions, directions, and more. We get to use the very same thing that got us in this place to get us out. With The Sweep, we're going to be sending directions to the subconscious mind that ask it to release those beliefs that aren't working for us. You can equate this to a focused meditation where we ask your subconscious mind to let old ideas be gently guided out and a new idea to be gently guided in.

We're going to use specific verbiage to do this. The Sweep is not a form of hypnosis, but it does use words that will relax the body and brain enough to allow us to change its programming. The phrase "I am now free …," which appears in almost every sentence, is key to the process. Freedom is a natural human desire, and it is counterintuitive, as humans, to resist it in any way. Since the subconscious mind resists so much, we are speaking the body's language here so that it works with us.

You might want to record this verbiage on your phone or other recording device so you can listen along to it and relax deeply while going through this process.

Just take it slow, really trying to sink into the words. If your mind wanders, it's okay. That can happen sometimes with this technique. Additionally, your wandering mind may be a sign that there are energies associated with those thoughts trying to clear. Just let go and allow the process to unfold.

Yawning, sighing, getting the chills, feeling emotional, burping, or stomach gurgling are all good signs of release. Just slow down to let your body process if you need to at any point. There is no need to hurry.

**Step 1: Connect with Your Inner Being or Higher Power**—I usually have clients place their hands over their heart to connect to their inner being or higher self. However, if you feel called to place your hands somewhere else, perhaps over an area that needs healing, feel free to do that instead.

**Step 2: Repeat The Sweep Verbiage**—Simply repeat the following script slowly, taking breaks if you feel like you need time to process (yawn, take a deep breath, etc.). Make sure you do not rush through this, as you need to do it in a way that feels inviting and safe to the subconscious mind.

*Even though I have this _____ (state the belief), I acknowledge it's no longer working for me.*

*I give my subconscious full permission to help me clear it, from all of my cells in all of my body, permanently and completely.*

*I am now free to thank it for serving me in the past.*

*I am now free to release all resistances to letting it go.*

*I am now free to release all ideas that I need this in order to stay safe.*

*I am now free to release all ideas that I need it for any reason.*

*I am now free to release all feelings that I don't deserve to release it.*

*I am now free to release all conscious and subconscious causes for this belief.*

*I am now free to release all conscious and subconscious reasons for holding on to it.*

*I am now free to release all harmful patterns, emotions, and memories connected to it.*

*I am now free to release all generational or past-life energies keeping it stuck.*

*All of my being is healing and clearing this energy now, including any stress response stored in my cells.*

*Healing, healing, healing.*

*Clearing, clearing, clearing.*

*It is now time to install _____ (insert a belief that is the opposite of whatever you just released; for example, if the belief was "I am too damaged to heal," you could install "I am perfectly able to heal.").*

*Installing, installing, installing.*

*Installing, installing, installing.*

*And so it is done.*

When you are finished, take a few big, deep breaths.

**Step 3: Check In**—It's a good idea to use your muscle testing to confirm that you cleared the belief completely. Simply state the belief again, in its original form, and see whether your body still resonates with it (and needs a little more work) or it's no longer true for you (wahoo!).

If, for some reason, the belief didn't clear completely, don't be alarmed. You can just repeat The Sweep again and retest. This process can take a few times of slow, deliberate intention and focus. Alternatively, you can move on to use Chakra Tapping, which you'll learn next. This will help you continue clearing the layers. Each belief will be different and will clear differently, too.

*Tip:* The Sweep can also be used effectively for clearing layers of energy contributing to symptoms. You might want to experiment with this. Instead of inserting a belief into the verbiage, you might use something like this: *Even though I have this _____ (insert symptom, fear, emotion, or anything else), I acknowledge it's no longer working for me.* Then revise the wording to fit your specific focus. I use this technique to clear pretty much everything, whether it be a certain emotion I'm feeling strongly in the moment or a thought that feels stuck in my head.

## Chakra Tapping

Chakras, the spinning energy centers in the body, hold old stories and experiences in their energies. Their energies are directly tied to early childhood programming and conditioning, which makes them a great access point into harmful beliefs.

During my own healing, I started off using Emotional Freedom Technique to clear beliefs. This worked quite well. However, as I discovered more about the chakras and how they hold our energetic history within them, I began to explore using them to clear beliefs. Remember, beliefs are really just old stories, usually from earlier in our lives.

With this connection between beliefs and the chakra system in mind, I wondered if it might make sense to tap directly on the chakras instead of using EFT tapping points, which are associated with the meridian system. I tried it, and voilà! I fell in love. I felt like I often got a deeper clearing than with EFT while also giving those ever-so-important chakras some attention too. We're going to use a very similar process to what you learned for EFT, but we'll tap on chakra points to address the chakra system instead. Easy!

## Chakra Review and Tapping Points

We covered the chakras in chapter 6, but let's briefly review them as a reminder of how these old stories might have found energetic homes in various places in your body. For each chakra that we review here,

I've also added its tapping point so you'll know exactly where to tap for this technique in order to clear.

*Crown (Seventh) Chakra*—Located on the top of the head, the crown chakra symbolizes spirituality and your connection to a higher power. It is tied to the energy of knowing you can trust life, that you are being taken care of and guided. The focus of the crown chakra is to help you connect with your purpose in life and your connection to a higher source. **Tapping Point:** top of the head.

*Third Eye or Brow (Sixth) Chakra*—This chakra is located directly between the eyebrows. It represents intuition, imagination, reflection, and the ability to see things for what or how they are (interpretation). Its focus is vision and inner guidance. **Tapping Point:** in between the eyebrows (be extra gentle with this point).

*Throat (Fifth) Chakra*—Located in the center of the throat, this chakra is about expression, communication, and truth. Its focus is communication and expression. **Tapping Point:** front of the throat.

*Heart (Fourth) Chakra*—The heart chakra is located in the center of your chest. It is linked to love, intimacy, forgiveness, and the ability to send and receive love. It's also responsible for your heart's desires and helping you manifest those desires. Its focus is love, relationships, and inner healing. **Tapping Point:** in the middle of the chest, at your heart's center.

*Solar Plexus (Third) Chakra*—The solar plexus chakra, located just below the sternum, governs your sense of personal power, including your personal choices and actions in the world. Its energy is tied to self-confidence, self-esteem, and a feeling of being in control of your life. It stores your judgments and opinions about the world and yourself. Its focus is personal power and a positive mentality. **Tapping Point:** right under the sternum at your solar plexus.

*Sacral (Second) Chakra*—The sacral chakra, also referred to as the womb chakra, is located in the pelvis behind the navel. It relates to your creativity and feelings and is also linked to childlike joy. It represents sexuality and is tied closely to your stories and conditioning from childhood. Its focus is feelings, creativity, and joy. **Tapping Point:** just below the belly button.

*Root (First) Chakra*—The root chakra is located at the base of the spine. It represents your feelings of safety and survival. It's connected to early childhood beliefs, money, and identity. It deals with issues of abandonment, unworthiness, and insecurity. Its focus is safety, security, and survival. **Tapping Point:** lower sacrum or top of your thighs. (Using flat hands to gently slap your thighs, pretend you are continuously motioning for a puppy to come sit on your lap.)

After creating and using a set-up statement, which I'll walk you through again, you're going to tap through all of the previous points. Starting at the top of your head, you're going to tap and talk about the belief in as much detail as possible. If you discovered earlier through muscle testing that you needed to identify and clear a specific unprocessed experience, you should have flipped back to chapter 7 and done that. You can just work with the belief itself now.

As you go through this process, just pretend you're telling me, or your best friend, about the belief. Tell us how the belief makes you feel, memories you recall that may be connected to it, where you feel it in your body, and whatever else comes to mind. This will be familiar to you from the process of Emotional Freedom Technique that you already learned.

Note: If this is a generational belief, talk about where you think it came from, how it makes you feel, and any other details that spontaneously come up. Guessing and pondering out loud will work quite well for this process.

**Step 1: Create a Set-Up Statement**—Just as with Emotional Freedom Technique, we're going to start by creating a set-up statement. Remember, the set-up statement has two parts.

*Even though _____ (state the experience), I _____ (insert a positive idea).*

For the first part, you will simply insert the belief. For the second part, you will insert any positive statement to balance the set-up. You are essentially telling yourself that even though something bad happened (first part), there is a positive, too (second part).

**First part of statement:** *Even though* _____ *(state the belief), ...*

**Second part of statement:** *..., I* _____ *(insert a positive idea).*

As a reminder, here are some positive ideas you could use for the second part of the set-up statement:

- *I completely love and accept myself.*
- *I can relax now.*
- *I am okay anyway.*
- *I choose to release it.*
- *I give my subconscious permission to let it go now.*

Here's an example belief that I took from that long list earlier in this chapter:

*I'll end up alone if I heal (people only stick around because I'm sick).*

The full set-up statement for this belief could be:

*Even though I'll end up alone if I heal, I choose to release it anyway.*

**Step 2: Use Your Set-Up Statement While Tapping the Karate Chop Point**—Now you'll continuously tap on the karate chop point while saying the full set-up statement three times.

**Step 3: Tap Through the Rest of the Points**—Next, you're going to simply tap through the rest of the chakra points and talk about the belief. You can use a mix of stating the belief, talking about how you feel about it, wondering aloud how you might have gotten it, and more. This is essentially a bit of improv!

The simple goal is to focus on this belief so we can bring up the energy and clear it. It's okay to temporarily focus on the belief; it will not get embedded in your system just by acknowledging it. In fact, this is essential to releasing it. The words you use are not at all important for this first round. You just need to talk about it and bring it up.

To show you how this could go, let's use the example belief of *I'll end up alone if I heal.* Here is what that might look like:

### Round 1

**Top of head:** *I might end up alone.*

**Third eye:** *I haven't taken care of myself in so long, I don't remember how!*

**Throat:** *If no one helps me, I'll just get sick again.*

**Heart:** *It reminds me of when I turned eighteen and Mom said, "You're on your own!"*

**Solar plexus:** *I'm so frustrated that this is keeping me from healing.*

**Belly button:** *But I believe that if I get better, people will just ditch me.*

**Top of thighs:** *Part of me really believes I can't take care of myself.*

### Rounds 2, 3, and 4

Now you are going to repeat what you did in round 1 for several more rounds. Just like the venting process we used in EFT, you're essentially doing the same thing here. It's okay, and sometimes even beneficial, not to use the same exact words and phrases from the first round. Just go with whatever comes up naturally.

**Step 4: Break**—Take a tapping break and a few deep breaths. Yawn or sigh if you need to. This little bit of time will help your body process the energy and release it fully.

**Step 5: Last (5th) Round**—Finally, you want to tap through the points one more time while stating a positive affirmation that you'd like to take in. This should ideally oppose the energy of what you just cleared. Example: *It's safe to heal now.* Alternatively, you can use the phrase *healing* at each tapping point.

**Step 6: Check In**—You may very well have cleared the belief by now. Using muscle testing, simply state the belief again in its original form, and see whether your body still resonates with it (meaning it's still there) or if it's no longer true for you (meaning it's cleared).

If it is clear, then you can high-five yourself now. If not, that's okay too, as it often takes some persistence. You can repeat the chakra-tapping process a few more times. If you're comfortable with muscle testing, you can make it easy for yourself and ask your body what technique would be best to repeat for full clearing, The Sweep or Chakra Tapping. Once I got confident with muscle testing, this became an essential part of my process: asking my body just what technique would be most beneficial for me instead of guessing. I do that in client sessions now, too.

*Tip:* Chakra Tapping and Emotional Freedom Technique can often be interchangeable. Both techniques are great, one working with the meridian system and the other with the chakra system. It's a fun exercise to play around with alternating these to see what works best for you, and when.

You can tap on chakras to move any type of stagnant energy. Just use gentle tapping for several minutes on any chakra that you feel might be blocked, according to what you learned in chapter 6.

## A Final Note on Harmful Beliefs

While we've been focusing on clearing harmful beliefs that directly oppose your healing goals, there is another type of belief I'd like to point out. This type of belief, while maybe not in direct opposition to your healing, can cause enough of a stress reaction in your body that it is hindering it. That means your stressful relationship with or reaction to this type of belief is not beneficial for you.

Here are some examples of these types of beliefs:

- *Mom loves my brother more than me.*
- *I'll always be behind with my career.*
- *I'm stupid.*
- *I'll always be alone.*
- *Everyone always excludes me.*
- *I am damaged.*
- *I am always left behind.*
- *I am always last.*
- *If I feel my feelings, I'll die.*
- *If I feel my feelings, I'll never be happy again.*
- *I'm only safe when others are happy.*
- *I need permission to be who I really am.*
- *Something bad will happen if I express my feelings.*

Do you see how believing these things wouldn't be conducive to creating a healing environment? These types of beliefs may not create the same type of healing self-sabotage that we've been focusing on so far, but they are definitely not beneficial. Even if the belief is actually factual at the moment, such as "I don't make enough money," using the technique to clear the stress reaction around that belief will do wonders for you.

Remember, your reality is directly linked to your beliefs, so it can seem like a bit of a chicken-or-the-egg scenario as to what came first—but changing one can change the other! We are in a constant energy dance with the universe, always co-creating. Our beliefs are an incredible part of that dance. A great exercise in finding non-beneficial beliefs is to take a hard look at your reality. Because our reality is a reflection of our beliefs, we can easily find what we believe just by looking at our lives. If your reality is that you don't have enough money or love, you might have a belief that "there isn't enough to go around" or "I'll always be poor." If it feels like nothing goes right for you, you may have the belief that "good things happen to everyone except me." In other words, if you see a certain pattern show up in your reality, you may have the belief to match it.

I want to share one final story with you to demonstrate how clearing beliefs can really transform your well-being for the long haul.

When I came back from India after nine weeks of stem cells, I was pumped with messages from my doctors that became beliefs for me, causing great stress. They kept telling me that if I caught a cold or the flu, did "too much," ate sugar, or was under any stress, I would relapse. This is a very common statement or belief associated with Lyme disease. However, this became a stress in and of itself for me. *I can't handle stress. I'll get sick if I catch a cold. Relapse is inevitable.*

I am sure, knowing what I know now, that those beliefs affected my physical body. I now know this, though. Once you do the inner work and strengthen your being at a core level, which includes changing your reactions to stress (remember, the stress isn't the issue; it's your relationship with it), you will not be the fragile person you might have felt to be before. It's essential to update your mental records about these types of inner dialogue and beliefs so that you do not continue to perpetuate a pattern that is no longer true or necessary for you.

After I healed completely using energy therapy, I went through many difficult experiences in my life, including the death of several family members in a very short time period. But I was okay anyway. My system remained in balance because of all the work I had done. I made sure to acknowledge and process difficult emotions as they arose, and I didn't hold the belief that these experiences would take me down. I am convinced this is why I never relapsed even during some of the most challenging times of my life.

My response to these types of experiences had totally changed from the days when I was perhaps an inch away from sliding backward at all times, and so did the belief that this would become my reality. You're well on your way to that freedom, too. Just keep in mind always that you can be okay no matter what.

### Chapter Nine

# Transform Unhealthy
# Emotional Patterns

*You will find that it is necessary to let things go;*
*simply for the reason that they are heavy.*
—C. JOYBELL C.

Well-being comes from being who you really are and accepting your-self in that space, no matter what. There are several unhealthy life patterns that I consider "spirit squashers," which make that level of love, acceptance, and well-being very difficult to achieve. Here is a question I get often and want to address before we start talking about unhealthy emotional patterns: "If we are supposed to love and accept ourselves for who we are, why are we trying to change so much about ourselves?"

The answer is simple: We don't want to change who we are, but we do want to change anything in our lives that isn't working for us. We don't need to keep unhealthy patterns that have become part of our lives but are not part of our best selves. For example, I'm an impatient person by nature sometimes. When clients hear me say that, they wonder why I don't "fix it." But the truth is, that's just part of who I am, and it's okay with me. It doesn't inhibit my quality of life. I don't want to spend my whole life nitpicking my personality. I want to spend my life living in the freest way possible, accepting all that I can about my-self and changing only what really hinders my quality of life.

You may have practiced some of them for a very long time—quite possibly, for your whole life. They are probably threaded into your being to such a great degree that when you read them, you might not even recognize they don't *have* to be that way. But that's the beauty here. You can change any pattern that's not working for you, no matter when you may have learned it.

These unhealthy life patterns include the following:

- Draining vocabulary
- Negative self-talk
- Victim mentality
- Taking things personally
- Negative thought loops

If you resonate with any of these patterns, you'd be wise to sit quietly and ask yourself if you're really ready to let go now. Don't beat yourself up if you're not. They can be scary to change. However, if you get a gentle nod that it's time to "shift that shit" (as I often say to myself), then I'm ready to help you.

With each pattern, where applicable, I'll be offering you some ideas of what types of unprocessed experiences (chapter 7) and harmful beliefs (chapter 8) might be connected to them. Then you will be able to clear them using the techniques you learned in those chapters. At the end of this chapter, I'll also share a brand-new technique (3 Hearts Method) for clearing emotional energy. I've waited to introduce it until now, as I didn't want to overwhelm you with too many techniques at once. Once you learn it, you may want to combine the 3 Hearts Method with the other practices, or use it independently.

## Draining Vocabulary

My motto: *Be careful what you tell yourself because you're always listening.* Oh, ain't it the truth? While this definitely pertains to self-talk, it also applies to our general day-to-day language with others, and that affects how we feel just as much. Here, we are going to discuss both types of language: vocabulary that we use every day in conversations with others and our own internal self-talk.

When I became convinced of the immense power of the mind-body healing approach, I also became aware of every facet of myself that wasn't in alignment with helping me heal. I then began to see phrases and sentences that I spoke as either reaching toward where I wanted to be or reaching away from it. With that new perspective, I came up with several words that I chose to ditch from my vocabulary, and I invite you to consider doing the same.

The only thing you need to do to change outdated language patterns is become aware of when you're using them, and immediately stop. Just don't go there. These everyday language patterns are simply a habit, and you can undo them by forming a new habit and using better-feeling language.

*Busy*—This implies having a great deal to do. Busyness is an addiction. Our society prides itself on being busy—it means we're doing, making things happen, and being "useful." The common excuse of "I'm too busy to..." implies you don't have a choice. Non-truth. Not having a choice is stressful. Choosing from a place of what feels good is calming.

Instead, try *engaged*. "I'm really engaged this week, so I choose to dedicate my free time to what I really want to do."

*Overwhelm*—This means to bury or drown beneath a huge mass; to overpower or crush. Yeah, this one just isn't pretty. Let's drop the *over* and stick with *whelmed*, which can be interpreted as "abundant." Nothing can crush us, and telling our body all day that we're "overwhelmed" isn't a healthy message to send it. You'd never even think of saying "I'm being crushed" over and over to yourself, would you?

Instead, try *whelmed*. "I'm whelmed with an awesome full list of opportunities."

*Anxiety*—This is a feeling of uneasiness, typically about an imminent event or something with an uncertain outcome. The word *anxiety* doesn't say exactly how you feel. Using the general word of "anxiety" let's us off the hook of figuring out what's really there, and dealing with it. In my opinion, anxiety is buried emotion. Not using it will help you call yourself to the challenge of figuring out "what" is sitting beneath it just waiting to be acknowledged and processed.

Instead, try *emotional* or *uneasy*. This is neither negative nor positive. It just is. "I'm feeling emotional (or uneasy) and I want to figure out why."

*Chronic*—This word means persisting for a long time or constantly recurring. I'm all about aligning with beliefs that promote what we really want. The word *chronic* essentially implies this issue or thing does not have an end in sight. Using the word and attaching its label to you isn't any way of aligning with the belief that it will pass sooner rather than later, right?

Instead, try *experiencing*. This one works as a substitute perfectly, and does not at all imply that you plan to hang onto it for a long time or as a recurring event. "I am experiencing this _____ (challenge)."

*Should*—This word is used to indicate obligation, duty, or correctness, typically with someone's actions. *Should have* implies a mistake, that something was done wrong and there is someone to blame. It's easier to be easy on ourselves when we're not declaring an action as "wrong," but rather simply looking at what the other side of the coin could have shown us.

Instead, try *could have*. This is a baby step in the right direction. *Could have* implies a choice, and choices always come from being in a good place. If one choice doesn't work out, we get to choose, and choose again. "I could have done this or that."

*My* _____ *(insert name of challenge)*—While possessives are necessary in the English language, it's wise not to claim anything that you don't actually want to be yours, like emotions, diseases, or other challenges. Examples of this include *my cancer, my anxiety, my anger issues,* and so on. These can all be rephrased with language that is relaxing to the body instead of stressful.

Instead, try the words *the* or *this*. Healthier rephrases include *the cancer* or *this cancer, the sadness I'm feeling*, or *the anger I'm experiencing*. All of these phrases support separation from the issue or the fleetingness of it, implying that it is moving through you or is not owned by you.

*I am* _____ *(insert emotion)*—There is such a fine line between *feeling* something and *being* something. Along the same lines as replacing the word *my*, *I am* is another phrase that implies ownership of things we may not necessarily want to claim.

Instead, try *feel*. "I feel sad." "I feel sick."

*Bonus Suggestion:* Although these things might not be something we typically think of as "language," it's wise to make sure email addresses, passwords, forum screen names, and so forth are not claiming energetic ownership over the very thing you don't want. This includes being *lymegirl, chronicfatigue4ever, anxietysurvivor*, or anything else in cyberspace. You cannot "be" something and separate from it at the same time.

One way to shift the pattern of using any of the draining vocabulary we've covered is to immediately correct yourself. Rephrasing it out loud, if you're comfortable, is a great way of "erasing" the energy that you just put out there. Or you can simply say something like "delete" or "oops!" in your head. That will help send a message to notify all those unconscious parts of you that it's time to reprogram your language.

### Energies to Consider Clearing

Another way to approach draining vocabulary is to look for beliefs or unprocessed experiences that cause you to use this language. For example, if you are hooked on the word *busy*, it might be beneficial to look at beliefs you have about being "too busy" to choose yourself and your own needs instead of everyone else's. What do you believe would happen if you did? Would someone be mad at you? Do you have a past experience in your history that gives this belief its roots?

## Negative Self-Talk

Imagine for a moment that our bodies obey each thing we tell ourselves as if it's a command. It does not filter or translate; it simply takes it in and acts. Now, the scary part is, you don't have to imagine. You are, with your internal self-talk, commanding your cells to believe or do as you say—either verbally or internally. Make sure you don't have a "shitty committee" in your brain running the show, okay? We need to give ourselves commands that align with healing. The only commands that align with healing are ones that remind us that we are worthy of healing because we rock, not suck.

After practicing a pattern of beating yourself up for so long, it would be almost impossible to instantly transform into a self-loving work of art, so take baby steps. Instead of aiming for thinking everything you do is golden, let's start by helping you be lighter with yourself and accepting your humanness. The goal is to laugh at yourself more and yell at yourself less.

### Accept Your Humanness

My approach for accepting my humanness came from something my dear friend Julia said to me in my twenties. I was telling her a story about someone in my life who hurt me. I was waiting with anticipation to hear an angry reaction, and for her to come to my rescue in defense. But what happened next changed my entire perspective, and how I judged not only others and their actions but my own as well. With almost no pause after my last sentence, she said calmly, "Well that sounds very human to me." In that moment, she rescued me from myself, and everything I judged before as either "good" or "bad," "right or "wrong," suddenly slipped into the singular category of "being human." Those words helped me take the first baby steps toward transforming the way I treated myself. When I caught myself judging, berating, or being critical of my experiences or myself, I threw my arms up and said, "Well, that was very human!" It made it difficult to judge something as right or wrong, because it was simply the truth. And how could I argue with that?

To this day, I use Julia's words in client sessions. Often clients nervously tell me they want to share something that they have never told anyone else before. And after they tell me, I say calmly, "Well, that sounds very human to me." The acknowledgment of being human is a miraculous little spark that brings peace and relief almost immediately. With that, I can feel their energy shift completely. And luckily for you, those words will forever remain available. Just remember, use often and apply liberally.

### Call It Out

This next little gem is a simple trick I used regularly to retrain myself away from a pattern of negative self-talk. As soon as I would recognize being lost in a loop of B.S. in my brain, I would call myself out on it. Because by now we all know better than to let that loop roll and gain any momentum, right? I'd say out loud, in my most fun and loving tone, "I call bullshit!" That's it. It's a light and silly way of holding yourself responsible for changing this pattern.

Remember, your body is always listening. If it listens to something long enough, it will start to believe it. It did when you told it sucky things for all those years, and it can when you send the opposite message, too.

### Energies to Consider Clearing

While using draining vocabulary in your day day-to-day is typically just a bad habit and can be altered consciously, negative self-talk can run much deeper.

It may be beneficial to clear past experiences where...

- you made a mistake or choice you can't forgive yourself for.
- others told you negative things about yourself.
- you felt that you embarrassed yourself.

Further, you may be holding harmful beliefs that are driving that negativity toward yourself. Here are a few examples:

- *I need to punish myself.*
- *Being mean to myself will motivate me to be better.*
- *I shouldn't be forgiven for the past.*
- *I owe it to others to be perfect.*

## Victim Mentality

This is a pattern that I had somehow mastered, although it took years for me to realize it. My personal pattern was fairly subtle, but once I saw it, boy, did I see it! I'll go so far as to say this pattern can be an addiction for some—the pattern of blaming outside circumstances, playing the part of "poor, pitiful me," or claiming little to no responsibility for one's life circumstances. The difficulty with identifying this pattern is that it shows up in so many ways, and they aren't always obvious.

This pattern often manifests as talking about the illness or challenge all the time, always bringing the conversation back to how you have been wronged: the doctors did you wrong, the disease is unfair, a person ruined your life, your past "did this" to you, and more. Of course, it's healthy to share experiences, but there is a fine line between sharing and putting yourself in a place of powerlessness. People with this pattern often perceive themselves as worse off than anyone else and need others to see them in that way, too. They seek confirmation from others that they have struggled more than their friends and family. They may have a need to be a hero, a survivor, that person who has "been through hell," sometimes feeling that this validates their worth. There is nothing shameful about the victim-mentality pattern. It's very common, but it's also extremely harmful.

Lyme disease, because it's highly controversial and not well understood by many, offered me the perfect opportunity to hold this pattern (and, later, to release it). Not only are there two camps of doctors, each professing a different truth about contraction, diagnosis, and treatment, but insurance companies often don't pay for the treatment that is recommended by physicians who specialize in Lyme disease. So there I was, not only bitten out of the blue by some horrible insect, but also now being told that the treatments my doctor recommended (sometimes in excess of thousands of dollars per month) would not be covered by my insurance. This left me feeling very frustrated. In the beginning, I shared this unfairness with those around me. I obsessively warned people about ticks, told them about the difficulty in getting diagnosed, and shared my treatment struggles. It felt good to have a place to direct the blame for my miserable situation.

However, as time went on, I realized that this energy was doing nothing but creating more helplessness and struggle. While perhaps all of the experiences that led me to this victim mentality and behavior were valid, my feeding of that energy by constantly engaging others in it, talking about it, and researching it was certainly not hurting the tick or the insurance companies. I was the one who was being hurt—by myself.

Suddenly I saw things clearly. I was making the unfairness worse by making Lyme disease more a part of my life than it had to be. I included it in both internal thoughts and external conversations. I let the perception that everyone and everything was against me take over. If you look at this pattern with a big ol' open heart, you will eventually realize that while you may have experienced wrongdoing once or even several times, every time you act from a place of victim energy, *you* are re-victimizing yourself. Chris Grosso, author of *Indie Spiritualist: A No Bullshit Exploration of Spirituality,* offers a question in his book that is fitting for this discussion. He writes: "Are we going to continue on autopilot, allowing our incessant negative thoughts and emotions to dictate our mental and emotional well-being? Or are we going to own our shit and take the power back?"

Releasing the victim mentality is all about taking our power back. It may not be easy, but it is your job, and until you are accountable for that job, you will not reach your full healing capacity.

Complaining, whether outright or subtly, is a victim pattern. It is a direction of energy toward what we do not want. We need to stop complaining, not because crappy things didn't happen or because they aren't horrible or upsetting, but because complaining is destructive. What message are we sending to our bodies—each organ and cell—when we align with the idea of being a victim? We must always consider, with each action and each word, what message we are sending ourselves.

Sharing my thoughts on victim energy is a conversation I have with many, many clients. Some immediately reject the idea that they are participating in this type of energy, and I've been there, so I understand this well. But for those who are ready, putting effort toward changing this pattern is full of great rewards.

I'll share an example with you. In a difficult session I had with Maggie, who I had been working with for about a month for a host of emotional challenges, I said to her: "I understand you are miserable and have had lots of things happen in your life that you wish never had, but you carry such enormous victim energy that I think it's a bigger block than anything else." I went on to explain to Maggie that in every session she was so focused on recalling things that weren't fair in her life and proving to me that they were so horrible and worse than her friends' problems that she was actually adding energy and weight to them. She was far more interested in blaming than clearing energy imbalances. I certainly expect clients to share with me what's not working in their lives so I can help, but this went far beyond sharing in that way. I couldn't even imagine how much she was doing this outside of sessions, too. No wonder she was constantly on the edge of panic.

It wasn't even just that Maggie was talking about her feelings, though; she was making her whole life about how wronged, sick, and abandoned she was. Maggie was not happy with me when I shared my observations, but after she had time to mull it over, she sent me an email. She explained that she had never realized she was giving off such a "poor me" energy and said she really wanted help with it. We then began focusing on that in sessions, and Maggie became more conscious of it on her own. She just didn't let herself go there anymore. Maggie's entire life changed when she changed this pattern. Her health made a huge turn in the right direction, she finally got into a living situation that was healthy for her, she stopped attracting friends who hurt her, and she got an incredible job—all things she admitted she never could have imagined could come from this change. But it was all because she stopped treating herself like a victim. Like Maggie, we all have a choice.

There is one simple question you can ask yourself to help determine which choice you are making: *Will this action, language, or behavior deplete my healing energy or fuel it?* That's it. New rule: If it will deplete it, delete it.

Consider making a pact with yourself: Don't have conversations (with yourself or others) that support this pattern. Simply refuse to let yourself go there. Instead, when you catch yourself talking about your life in a way that makes you feel powerless, sit quietly and try to figure out why you have a need to do this. Are you seeking support and confirmation? Do you need help but can't ask for it? Try instead to use this as an opportunity to clear energy around these issues.

### Energies to Consider Clearing

Often, there are unprocessed experiences lurking behind this victim mentality. It is wise to identify and clear experiences in your past that are contributing to this mindset.

These types of experiences might include experiences where…

- you felt like people didn't "pay for" the way something impacted you.
- you felt overpowered and had "no say."
- you feel like life wasn't fair to you.

Beliefs are also likely behind this pattern. Going to work on clearing beliefs that put you in a place of powerlessness will always be extremely helpful. Here are a few examples:

- *I can only move on if those who hurt me are sorry.*
- *Other people are responsible for fixing me/this issue.*
- *I need to blame others to feel secure.*
- *I need to be rewarded for what I've been through.*
- *Life isn't fair to me.*
- *I always get the short end of the stick.*

- *People owe me (sense of entitlement).*

## Taking Things Personally

We were all born as wonderful, self-centered works of art. As human beings, we tend to be self-focused, and that's okay a lot of the time. But it can get us into big trouble, too, because we tend to interpret everything as if it is personal. It's all too easy from our human vantage point to see the opinions and actions of others as direct reflections of our own wrongdoing.

I used to be the queen of "it's my fault" syndrome. If someone I loved or cared about seemed "off," I felt a heavy sense of fear that I had somehow inadvertently caused it. If someone seemed upset with me, I quickly jumped into action to fix it, at the expense of my poor, overburdened soul. To this day, I have no idea where this originated. Growing up, I was never blamed or ridiculed, although now I can definitely see my mom's own pattern of self-blame for things.

It wasn't until my early twenties that I thought to examine this pattern in my life. Most of us think that the whole wide world revolves around us, and that's just a big ol' problem. Becoming aware of how this affected me changed how I perceived everything. Up until then, I lived a life being paranoid that others were angry with me, or upset *because* of me. But for the first time, it occurred to me that the world doesn't revolve around me at all. I began to see that each of us reacts from our own emotional space—of simply having a bad day, feeling insecure, being frustrated with someone else perhaps, and so on.

My days of taking things personally started to change ever so slowly. When I would fear that I had upset somebody or I would become angry because of how I thought they were treating me, I would ask myself, usually while laughing, "What makes you think that the whole world revolves around you?"

Let's do a quick exercise here. Look back at some of your recent personal interactions—times when someone in your life seemed grumpy or irritated. How did they make you feel? Did you assume you had done something wrong? Did you try to fix things immediately? Did you apologize when people were being impatient with you? If so, you likely had the mindset that it was all about you. This can cause us to tiptoe around others and be afraid to be our true selves. And we already know what a big impact that can have on us, right? That's why this is a very important pattern to work on.

### Forest Fire Visualization

I also use the visualization of a burning forest fire when I'm having difficulty with taking things personally. I imagine the person whom I am being upset by as a burning fire in a large wooded area. In this visualization, I draw a circle around the fire with a stick. I then know that I can be anywhere in that forest (symbolic of my own life and my own energy field) and be safe from the heat and sparks. I allow the fire (symbolic of the person in this specific situation) to be angry or do whatever it needs to do to burn out or dissolve. However, I don't allow myself to be affected. This is very helpful for me in staying grounded when others are upset, either in general or specifically with me.

With the pattern of taking things personally, it's very helpful to ask yourself, "Where could this pattern have come from?" In other words, "Where did I get the idea that I was responsible for everyone else and how they feel?"

### Energies to Consider Clearing

Unprocessed experiences from your past could be playing a direct role in this pattern of taking things personally. You might want to think back to experiences where…

- you felt blamed or shamed.
- you perceived that someone else's happiness was your responsibility.

As always, harmful beliefs are likely contributing to this pattern as well. Here are some examples of harmful beliefs to consider releasing:

- *Something is inherently wrong with me.*
- *When someone else is unhappy, it's my fault.*

- *I am always wrong.*
- *Keeping the peace is my job.*
- *It's my job to fix things for others.*
- *If I'm rejected, it means there is something wrong with me.*

## Negative Thought Loops

It can be easy to get stuck in a negative thought loop, which not only makes us feel a little crazy but also causes stressful reactions in our body, which can show up as symptoms.

As we know now, thoughts are pure energy. This next technique, Throwing Stones, is one that was created during a time of desperation for me. It is based on "throwing" energy from the body. It's a great disrupter of unhealthy thought patterns.

A few years ago and for no obvious reason whatsoever, right before a trip to the infamous and spirited city of Sedona, Arizona, I started to feel extremely unsettled. I was flooded with fear and uneasiness, which made me want to jump out of my own skin. Negative thoughts were looping around in my brain at what seemed like warp speed.

People travel from all over to visit Sedona and, specifically, its vortexes, which are thought to have highly concentrated energies conducive to healing. Sedona has been known as a sacred place for hundreds of years. As we prepared for the trip, I used all my best tricks, but in true Amy style, they weren't working instantly. They do work extremely well for me, but sometimes not as fast as I'd like. Sedona, a place known for healing, turned out to be, for me, just a place where I was having a serious freak-out. Very spiritual, right? I was in a location where miracles are known to happen, and I didn't want to leave my hotel room. I couldn't stop crying.

After a few days, though, I surrendered to what I was feeling and stopped fighting it so hard. I knew I just had to let all of the energy work do its thing. Something inside of me shifted, as often happens when we stop fighting so hard. I calmed down just enough to try to enjoy a short hike along a beautiful creek. The water was dotted with different-size boulders. While sitting on one of the giant ones for a rest, I dipped my still-shaky hands into the water to play with some of the smaller rocks. That's when I had a thought: What if I could "throw" or "wash" away the energy of whatever was coming up for me and send it hurling down the creek?

With each rock I picked up, I closed my eyes and imagined transferring a single thought, feeling, or emotion I had into it. I said a silent statement to the rock, asking it to please "carry away the energy" of each one: fear of what was happening, anger, uncertainty, nausea, the feeling of "not being good enough to fix this," and more. And then I threw the rock into the rushing water, watching it skip along the bottom until it was gone from my sight. One by one, I went through this process: assigning each rock an energy I no longer wanted, throwing it, and feeling my energy come back into balance. Energetically, I was transferring the feelings, thoughts, and emotions into those rocks to be carried away and washed clean. I felt massive relief from this process, and you can too.

### Throwing Stones

This is easy to do and you don't have to use rocks. You can use coffee beans, pebbles, snowballs, or anything else that won't hurt the earth if you toss it into a body of water. You can also use a bucket of water if you don't have access to a beach, pond, or other body of water.

When you have a decent little pile, pick them up one by one, assigning each one a thought or emotion you'd like to release. Simply focus on infusing that thought or emotion into the rock or other object. Take your time, but when you're ready, throw the object into the water using as much force as is comfortable, and let yourself release all that is associated with it.

This had already become one of my favorite techniques when I read an article about a similar concept. In a study at Ohio State University,[15] researchers found that when people wrote down their thoughts on a piece of paper and then threw the paper away, they mentally discarded the thoughts as well.

---

15. Jeff Grabmeier, "Bothered by Negative, Unwanted Thoughts? Just Throw Them Away," *Ohio State University* (Nov. 26, 2012), http://researchnews .osu.edu/archive/matthoughts.htm.

I believe this works as an energy technique because we are signaling to the subconscious mind to release the energy of the thought or emotion. So throw to your heart's content. All you have to lose is some energy that you didn't need anyway.

### Energies to Consider Clearing

Negative thought loops often stem from a belief or unprocessed experience that we haven't let go of. In order to release this, it's helpful to pay attention to those thoughts and address the core of them. What are you ruminating about? Is it an experience that can be cleared? Is it something you believe that's creating the negativity? Digging deeper into these thoughts can produce big, positive shifts.

## 3 Hearts Method

You've learned four main techniques up to this point, including Thymus Test and Tap, Emotional Freedom Technique, The Sweep, and Chakra Tapping. As I mentioned earlier, these techniques can be used to help you release the various unhealthy emotional patterns you've learned about in this chapter. The *3 Hearts Method* is another technique that I consider to be very important. It's the fifth (and final) main technique you'll learn.

The 3 Hearts Method was fed to me through some higher guidance during a difficult time. I was lying on the couch one night, my head hanging off the ottoman (a typical pose for me), and I spontaneously began tracing, with my hands, three upside-down hearts on my face. It almost seemed involuntary. I had no idea what I was doing, but I could feel energetically that I was most definitely doing something.

As I started to explore and use this new technique, it proved to be extremely powerful for releasing stored emotional energy associated with those incessant negative thoughts. While emotional processing happens in the brain, the expression of emotion is limited primarily to the face. Muscle movements that happen under the skin cause expressions. Certain facial expressions are associated with specific emotions. And emotions, as we know, are just energy. Because our cells and muscles have "memory," it is logical that some of the energy that causes negative thinking could easily become stored in the place of the most expression.

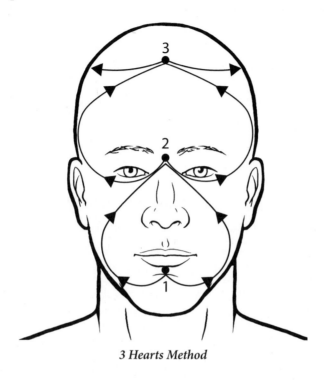

**3 Hearts Method**

The heart shape, symbolic of love, has an extremely high healing vibration. When we trace lines around the eyes and mouth, we are addressing the major emotionally expressive areas of the face. We are essentially "erasing" or "tracing over" whatever is behind the negative thoughts, with love. It is critical that the hearts be traced upside down so the "point" is always directing the old energy away from the body. With the third heart in the sequence, we are specifically tracing it around the head where emotions are processed and then finishing the sequence at the back of the head. Here again, the direction of the point is crucial, because we are sending the energy behind us, which is symbolic of moving those experiences and associated emotions into the past. This is where, in the energetic body, memories and thoughts—even negative ones— are stored in a healthy way.

In order to demonstrate this technique, I'll walk you through it using the example of a negative thought loop. Later, I will give you some tips on revising the 3 Hearts Method for clearing other energies, such as unprocessed experiences and harmful beliefs.

**Step 1: Rate Your Intensity**—Close your eyes and focus on the negative thoughts. On a scale of 0–10, give it a rating as far as how intense it feels for you, 10 being the strongest. If you can locate where you "feel" it in your body, also take note of that. It doesn't matter where you are at this moment; it's just good to have an idea of your starting point so you can gauge your progress as you clear.

If you have many upsetting thoughts and they're not just on one topic, you can let them all run through your mind, or you can focus on them one by one and go through this process for each thought pattern. You may have to try it both ways to see what works best for you.

**Step 2: Trace the Hearts**—As shown in the 3 Hearts Method illustration, keep your eyes closed and your focus on the upsetting thoughts as you trace, with medium pressure, three upside-down hearts on your face, as shown in the illustration. Use both hands. You will do the same movement on each side of your face simultaneously.

While you'll be tracing the hearts three at a time (this will be one "round"), you will want to continuously trace for four rounds, or a total of twelve hearts. I don't have a logical explanation for why we trace a total of twelve hearts, but through much muscle testing I discovered this was the magic number!

For the first heart, start with all your fingertips at your bottom lip point. Drag your fingers down toward your chin, around, and up your jawline, finishing at the second point—the bridge of your nose. For the second heart, starting at the bridge of your nose, scoop down around the eyes and up to the top center of your forehead where your hairline is. For the final heart, use a similar scooping motion down your forehead and then back along the sides of your head and past your temples, ending in a point at the back of the head. All three hearts should be traced consecutively in one fluid motion.

You want to really sink into the issue you are trying to clear. Let all the emotion come up, and allow yourself to review the issue in your head, noticing any details of the experience.

**Step 3: Check In**—Take a break, open your eyes, and take some big, deep breaths. Close your eyes and reassess how strong the negative thoughts are now. Do they bother you any less? Do you feel any more detached? Re-rate your thoughts on a scale of 0–10 to gauge their intensity.

**Step 4: Keep Going**—Repeat the process for several more minutes. You can continue this as long as you'd like, taking a break after every few rounds and making sure to take deep breaths and give your body time to process the energy.

With negative thought loops, it can often take a bit of time to notice a shift. You may want to just go about your day and see how things play out. With negative thought loops, I'll often wonder if the clearing has done anything, but then later I'll suddenly become aware of how much it has actually helped.

While this technique may seem too simple (yes, I've actually had that complaint!), it's extremely effective. Don't worry that it's "too easy to work." This is good practice in letting life be easy.

*Tip:* Remember that most unhealthy emotional patterns are linked to harmful beliefs or unprocessed experiences. For example, if you can't stop thinking about that mean thing your boss said to you last week, you would benefit from working on that experience, or earlier experiences that you were reminded of with that one. Or perhaps it would be beneficial to identify and clear a belief that is creating a trigger for you, such as "I am worthless at work." In addition to using techniques that you already know can address unprocessed experiences (EFT) and beliefs (Chakra Tapping), you can explore using the 3 Hearts Method to clear them.

To use the 3 Hearts Method for unprocessed experiences, simply alter steps 1 and 2 to focus on an unprocessed experience instead of specific negative thoughts. Try to use the glass-capsule analogy that we talked about earlier, making sure to focus on all of the details (sights, sounds, smells, and more) connected to that experience.

To use the 3 Hearts Method for beliefs, use a similar process to Chakra Tapping, but instead of tapping the chakra points, trace the three hearts. Remember to ask through muscle testing—just as you would when clearing any belief—if you need to go back and find an unprocessed experience to work with first. If not, you can use verbal cues like you did for Chakra Tapping as you trace the hearts, or you can just try focusing on the belief itself without saying anything at all. Again, make this method your own.

Next, we're going to talk about a serious game-changer: addressing fear.

### Chapter Ten

# Address the Real F-Word (Fear)

*Each of us must confront our own fears, must come face to face with them. How we handle our fears will determine where we go with the rest of our lives.*

—JUDY BLUME, *TIGER EYES*

When people ask me, as they often do, if I had to choose one thing that contributes to illness the most, I immediately tell them about the real F-word: Fear. Fear is not bad nor evil, but we have come to use it in all the wrong ways. There is nothing in our experience that is more constantly present and destructive than fear—an energy that is in direct opposition to wellness. Almost every single challenge can be traced back to the fear of ending up unsafe in this world (physically or emotionally).

In this chapter, you'll learn exactly what fear is, what causes it, and how it shows up in our lives. Then I'll share the two parts to addressing fear completely:

- *Clearing unprocessed experiences and beliefs that cause fear.* For each example of how fear might be showing up in your life, I'll offer ideas on what to clear related to it.

- *Using techniques to reprogram the fear response in your body.* Toward the end of the chapter, you will learn several wonderful tools to do that.

## What Fear Is

I believe that fear is a major common denominator, at some level, of every illness. Fear is perhaps the most practiced energy in our lives, from the time we are children and our well-meaning parents remind us to be careful, tell us not to talk to strangers, and convince us that Santa won't come if we're bad kids. Sometimes we even inherit fear from our parents. We live in a world of "fear feeders"—the media, well-meaning loved ones, people we look up to like doctors and advocates, and the list goes on and on. In every space of our lives, we are bombarded with the message that we need to fear.

The interesting thing is that the more fear energy you release, the more clearly you will see it governing those around you. Becoming less fearful may even trigger fear in others because it is so contradictory to what we've practiced our whole lives. In fact, we often make decisions from a place of fear. If you take a minute to think of all your actions and decisions that are fear-based, it probably won't take long to see how much of your life is being driven by fear. This includes taking a job because we're scared we won't get something better, listening to a doctor only because we're afraid not to, not speaking our truth because we're afraid of losing a loved one, and more. Fear can show up in its most aggressive form linked to matters of survival: relationships, money, and health.

In many cases, except in actual dangerous situations, fear is just energy with no merit. It is an indicator system that often malfunctions. Fear, in its most stripped-down form, is a response in the body that comes from feeling deeply unsafe in the world. This response is connected to the fight, flight, or freeze pattern, governed by the triple warmer meridian (aka your inner "papa bear"). We first learned about this earlier, in chapter 2.

## What Causes Fear

No matter how fear manifests in your life, there are usually two reasons it's hanging around.

First, your body holds some type of reason that the fear response is justified. This means that there is "evidence" in the form of harmful beliefs and unprocessed experiences.

Second, fear is an energy pattern. It has likely been replaying in your system for quite some time. So the fear response itself can be on auto-pilot. Knowing what causes it will help us to slowly clear this pattern. When you continue to clear unprocessed experiences and harmful beliefs causing fear, you are doing a big part of this work. You are clearing the root, or "evidence," of the fear. But you also need techniques to actually change the energetic pattern, too.

As the fear pattern plays out, you will learn to do very specific things to retrain or redirect it. You will need to work as a friend in partnership with that triple warmer meridian to do this, being patient and gentle.

We have to find a way to move through fear if we want enriched lives. It is something that is absolutely essential to clear in order to put our bodies into a state of ease.

## Common Ways That Fear Shows Up

You may be sitting there thinking, "I'm not a scared person." But fear is much bigger than simply being afraid. By spelling out specific ways that fear can show up in your life, I hope you will come to see just how important it is to work lovingly on this.

Just follow me. Let's peek inside that brain of yours and see if it lights up with any of these common fears. Then we'll go to work on releasing them.

### Fear of Being Who You Really Are

We've already talked a lot about this one, but I feel it's important to reiterate it here. I believe that our deepest fears as humans are the fears around being who we really are. And those are closely connected to the core fear that we started this discussion with: the fear of ending up *unsafe* in this world (physically or emotionally). The fear of being who we really are all boils down to these questions: *If I am who I really am, will I be unsafe? If I am who I really am, will I be unloved?*

During many of the exercises and practices in this book, whether through clearing unprocessed experiences, harmful beliefs, or other energies, you've simultaneously cleared energy around fear as well. Just stay aware of when triggers, roots, and energies connected to it pop up, and hold a strong intention that it's time now to move forward without it.

### Fear of Not Being in Control of Life

During my first weeks in India, as I learned more about myself, I became painfully aware of my fear of trusting in the flow of life. This country that so beautifully enveloped me in love and offered the opportunity for a renewed life also pushed me to the limits of my sanity.

The water temperature for showers was lukewarm at best. The streets were like tornadoes of dust swirling up into dense crowds of people who were sticking together from thick heat and humidity. There were dogs barking all night and horns honking around the clock without a second's reprieve. The cultural and language barriers led to a feeling of isolation that I'd never known before. I had a rat living in my hospital room with me. And most of the time I felt like I was slowly dying and there was no way to tell if the treatment was killing me or curing me.

I entered this country that runs on chaos and uncertainty ready to control and manipulate my life as I had always done, and it spit me out onto the broken pavement like a rejected piece of gum. India, as I eventually accepted, was not the place to try to be in charge. I tried, though.

The fear of not being in control of life comes from a worry that things will not be okay unless they happen exactly as we want or need, and/or an energy of lack—feeling there's not enough money, support, love, safety, or whatever, so we must take everything into our own hands in order to be okay. But what if we put our beautiful human egos aside for just a minute and considered it could all turn out okay? That the universe, God, or whatever higher source we resonate with, might have a plan to help us, if we allow it? I saw a massive shift in my being when I finally stopped fearing life. I learned to trust that if I was aligned with something and it was meant to be, it would find me in a hundred different ways.

Living with the fear of not being in control is like trying to paddle a canoe upstream instead of letting the current help you flow effortlessly downstream. The river is going where it's going and it's giving you a free ride, but you want to do it your way, right? You want to control every single stroke. You can find a million things to feel unsafe about. How long can you keep it up? Also, what if that elusive pot of gold you're paddling toward is actually in the other direction? You just have to let … go … of … the … freakin' … oars. Your body will thank you for it.

Learn and embrace, in the deepest core of your being, that you can handle anything that comes your way. You can survive. You can survive. You can survive. You can let go of the oars and be okay. Trying to control and manipulate your life's circumstances to force a feeling of safety will work only temporarily. Learning that you can be okay no matter what will create a true, lasting sense of security.

When you're feeling stuck about something, ask yourself, "Is this because I'm attached to making it how I think it should be instead of flowing along with how it actually is?"

I always say, *When you flow, you know.* In other words, if things are feeling too hard, you are probably pushing against life's current, and the fear of not being in control is likely hijacking your oars. It's always your call: Are you going to fight or flow?

### Energies to Consider Clearing
The following are examples of energies (which we've already learned about) that might be tied to the fear of not being in control.

*Unprocessed Experiences:*
- Times when you relaxed and something bad happened
- Times when someone blamed you for something getting messed up
- Times when you let someone down and they made you pay for it

- Times where you didn't have enough food, money, love, or security (controlling everything may seem like a good way to prevent those times from happening again)

*Harmful Beliefs:*
- *I'm only safe when I'm in control.*
- *Having money is the only way to feel safe.*
- *There's not enough to go around.*
- *I need to understand things to be okay with how they are.*
- *I can keep bad things from happening.*
- *I am unable to handle bad things.*

### Fear of Letting Others Be Who or How They Are

Trying to control other people's lives is sure to bring equal, or even greater, misery than trying to control your own. You can slice and dice and justify this one anyway you want, but it never, ever turns out well. It is simply not your responsibility or prerogative to change others.

Here are some examples of how we try to change others:

- Helping others when they don't want help
- Needing to help others to feel good about yourself
- Helping others even at the expense of your own well-being (having "obsessive-helperitis")
- Needing something from others (forgiveness, acknowledgment, or validation) for your own inner peace
- Needing others to behave in a certain way so you can relax or be happy

If any of these are familiar to you, you are draining your own energy. You are not allowed to stomp on anyone else's path for any reason. If we get brutally honest with ourselves, we often find that fears drive our need to control others. And these fears keep us from moving forward. We may have a fear that they will mess up and we'll have to pick up the pieces. We may fear if someone doesn't validate or take responsibility for how they've hurt us, it means we are to blame. We might fear that we won't get what we need from another person and end up hurt. We might be afraid that others will end up hurting themselves in some needless way. All of these things are understandable but not healthy.

When people love you, it will be in the way they know how. You can always focus on what they're not doing or how they're not being that makes your life uncomfortable. Maybe you feel they're not support-ive enough or compassionate enough or are always saying the wrong thing at the wrong time. But the fact is, you don't get to make that call. We all have the ability to love, but our capacity and willingness to do so is unique. To truly free yourself, you need to stop demanding that people behave in the ways you think they could or should. You can and certainly should remove yourself from any relationships that are unhealthy for you, but trying to change another person is a losing ap-proach.

When I was growing up, there was a rickety, doll-size antique red chair in my parents' house. The paint was chipped off, and the old, worn wood peeked through. My mom always loved anything that looked like it should have been retired years earlier, and despite how much we teased her about the chair, it traveled with us with each move, even after we all grew up and left home.

One day, while I was struggling not only with the decline of my health but also with a difficult personal relationship, my dad brought that rickety chair over to where I was sitting. By this time, I was all grown up. He put it in front of me and asked, "What is this?"

"A stupid red chair," I said.

He nodded in approval. "Now try to make it a big blue chair."

"Daaaaad," I begged. "I can't."

"Try harder. Make it blue."

"Dad, please …"

He egged me on. "Care more. Do more. Figure it out."

"I can't, I can't!" I finally screamed.

He sat down next to the chair. "Exactly, baby. You can't. This is a little red chair. It doesn't matter how much you want it to be blue or big and strong. It only has the capacity to be a little red chair, and nothing you can do will change that."

People are just like that chair, too. Since the red chair lesson, each time I come up against a situation in my life that frustrates me or makes me lose my sense of balance, I gently check in with myself to see whether I am trying to make a red chair blue. And guess what? I always am.

You must let people be who they are, not only for themselves but also for the sake of your little soul who just cannot be burdened with controlling another being. They may not be who you'd like them to be and they may even be jerks. But people can be jerks and you can be okay anyway.

## Communicate with Others' Higher Selves

When I find myself frustrated by my need to turn a red chair blue, I simply use something that my friend Scott taught me. I sit quietly and "send" my message to that person's higher self, which might be more willing to receive it. Can you think of someone who just won't listen to you or someone with whom it's impossible to communicate? Sit quietly with your eyes closed, imaging that person and setting the intention that the person's higher self or inner being will receive your message. Then simply say out loud what you need to say.

With this practice, I often feel instant relief. You may sense, like I do, that the energy is released from you and that you can now move forward, detached from "needing" to reach that person. People can and will change, indeed. But the danger comes when we need them or expect them to be someone else, simply for our own inner peace. Louise Hay has an affirmation that really drives this home: *I let go of all expectations. People, places, and things are free to be themselves, and I am free to be me.*

### Energies to Consider Clearing

For the fear of letting others be who and how they are, it's important to look at experiences and beliefs where you struggled because of somebody else. Here are some examples.

*Unprocessed Experiences:*

- Times when someone else's behavior made you unsafe
- Times when someone else, because of who they are, hurt you (inadvertently)
- Times when someone refused to hear your side of things and you felt rejected

*Hamful Beliefs:*

- *I'm only safe when I control others.*
- *It's my job to make others feel needed.*
- *I have to change others to feel safe.*

### Fear of Pain and Suffering

No one likes to experience pain and suffering. In fact, we spend much of our lives trying to avoid this. But believing that suffering is *bad* will cause more havoc in your life than actually experiencing it would. Suffering just *feels* bad while it's happening, and because of that, we fight it like the plague. But suffering also has a silver lining that never gets the credit it deserves. Suffering helps us grow and get to the next place in life. Let's face it: if not for suffering, we'd never stop in our busy lives to expand in ways that make us better.

Suffering can be a phenomenal steppingstone to somewhere better, physically, emotionally, or spiritually. Failed relationships get us to successful ones; illness helps us examine who we really are and what matters, when we might not otherwise; grief reminds us we are human and we *can* survive after inevitable loss; and the list goes on and on. Avoiding suffering does nothing but prolong the suffering.

Much unnecessary struggle in our lives comes not just from avoiding our own pain but from trying to avoid it or intercept it for others, too. Pain is a part of life, and it's an okay part. Avoiding or trying to fix another person's suffering instead of simply being present for it is a damaging emotional pattern.

Some examples of how the fear of suffering can manifest include feeling responsible for other people's feelings, feeling like you have the responsibility to make sure other's lives are going right, avoiding diffi-cult emotions, allowing yourself to be distracted from self-care, think-ing you know better for others than they do, and feeling like you have to save people from their own pain and mistakes.

It is important to remember that others are capable of working through their own suffering, just like you are. This is a necessary and beneficial part of life. When we overprotect another, we drain our own energy and rob that person of all the good that can come from fully allowing them their own experience.

We have an obligation in life not only to call ourselves to our own greatness, but to call others to theirs as well. And sometimes that hap-pens through outright painful experiences that are a normal part of life. Holding back our true selves is the single biggest act of betrayal we can perform. It puts a serious stress on our physical bodies, and we aren't doing a service to those we are trying to save, either.

This concept became clear to me when I was living in Delhi. When I was too sick to go outside of the hospital, I'd sit in front of a floor-to-ceiling sliding glass door at the front of the building. For weeks, I watched a man with no use of his legs pass the hospital. He used his arms to travel by scooting on his bottom, his fists powering movement along the pavement and dirt. His pants were torn to shreds and his hands were swollen with cuts.

I sunk into my chair wondering how he'd ended up like this and where he was going. Finally, I asked one of the doctors in the lobby why the man didn't have a wheelchair. "Oh, ma'am, it's too costly. It's approximately seventy-five dollars."

*Oh my goodness, this man is suffering for what seventy-five dollars could fix,* I thought. I decided I would buy this man a wheelchair. I asked the doctor to go outside and tell him about Operation Wheel-chair, as I was sure he wouldn't speak English and my Hindi knowl-edge was poor at best. The doctor hurriedly made his way down the stairs and crouched before the man as I watched in anticipation.

After a quick conversation, the doctor returned to the building and said, "He kindly declines your wheelchair offer." I was stunned. He explained that the man had asked what was wrong with the way he was. "He is fine this way, ma'am. This is his life and he is happy."

My stomach sunk and it felt like my Western ego had fallen out of my body and splattered on the floor. There was nothing wrong with this man in his eyes, just in mine.

While charity is obviously a very positive thing, this entire situation came from my own need to feel better about this man's life—which wasn't bothering him at all, from what I learned! From that day on, I redirected my focus from trying to save others and myself from suffering to becoming comfortable with suffering as a part of life. This helped me so much, and I bet this story could help you, too.

### Energies to Consider Clearing

Our beliefs about pain and suffering often come straight from how our parents feel about it. We also tend to learn about suffering from our religious upbringing. Here are some ideas on what to clear in relationship to fears around suffering.

*Unprocessed Experiences:*

- Times when you felt helpless while someone you loved suffered
- Times when you suffered and felt trapped in the suffering
- Times when someone around you made you feel like you deserved to suffer
- Times when you believe that suffering was punishment for something you did wrong
- Times when someone you loved (maybe a parent) avoided their own difficult feelings or distracted you from yours

*Harmful Beliefs:*

- *It's my job to spare others.*
- *Others can't handle pain like I can.*
- *No one should have to suffer.*
- *Someone has to suffer, so maybe it should be me.*

- *Suffering is bad.*
- *I will die if I suffer.*

### Fear of Not Being Perfect or Good Enough

My clients who experience the most intense emotional and physical symptoms are by far the ones who beat themselves up the most—usually about not being "perfect" or good enough (which means they have set a level of perfection they have to meet in order to be good enough). It's one and the same thing. Often the idea of being perfect (good enough) equates to being loved. We perceive that we need to be perfect to be loved. Imagine the fear of not being perfect as a mama duck: the leader. The additional fears of being judged and being rejected are just like little ducklings trailing behind. They are all stuck to each other like glue!

The fear of not being perfect may arise from your own expectations or because you internalize the expectations of others. It doesn't matter where the pattern originated, but it does matter that we spend as much time and energy as it takes to change it. We cannot be ourselves, embrace ourselves, and love ourselves when we are dominated by this fear. The two simply cannot coexist. We must learn to be easier on ourselves to be happy and healthy. And this is a big part of that.

What happens if we fear our imperfections so deeply that we continuously beat ourselves up for them? The research of Dr. Masaru Emoto demonstrates what happens to water molecules (just like those that make up a large percentage of your body) when they are exposed to negativity for a period of time. Even the simple exercise of writing negative words on paper and attaching them to the water bottles had a significant negative impact on the structure of the molecules. What if that energy of self-criticism is present inside of you constantly? If our minds are our leaders, how do we expect anything good to come from a leader who constantly judges him- or herself for not being perfect? Or a leader who accepts the criticism of others as truth? Exactly. We can't. We must love ourselves and ensure our bodies feel loved, despite all our messy imperfections, in order to invoke positive change. We don't have to be perfect at that either, but we do have to be the best we can possibly be.

The energetic frequency of love is believed to be the highest frequency that exists. The practice of loving ourselves despite our "imperfections" makes good sense for our overall well-being. And, as far as I know, love is impossible to get too much of, so it's a very safe approach.

Loving yourself is simply the act of treating yourself like a human being: being able to laugh at yourself, shrug your shoulders when you mess up, give yourself a break, and realize that you're perfectly fine just as you are. But in order to do that, you have to give up the gigantic assumption that you should, or even could, be perfect. And you must give up the need for others to see you as perfect, too.

Loving ourselves wells up from inside of us naturally, albeit sometimes slowly, like a pot that it seems will never boil. One minute there is nothing, and then the first bubble appears. But the first bubble is all it takes. And as we feel better in that space, we become less fearful of not meeting the perfectionist ideals that we placed such high value on before. We strive only to be ourselves, even if we are afraid that others won't like it.

We must allow ourselves to be human, full of imperfections, and embrace ourselves that way. Clearing unprocessed experiences and beliefs will help us do that more easily.

### Energies to Consider Clearing

Exploring and clearing "evidence" that fuels this fear of not being perfect is a great way to start. Here are a few ideas to get you thinking.

*Unprocessed Experiences:*

- Times when someone got mad at you for making a mistake
- Times when you perceived that your value was tied to being a "good girl" or "good boy"
- Times when someone punished you for not doing something their way
- Times where you feel you were judged or rejected for expressing yourself

*Harmful Beliefs:*

- *Bad things will happen if I'm imperfect.*
- *No one will like the real me.*
- *I have nothing to offer if I'm imperfect.*
- *I need to be perfect or I'll be rejected.*
- *I need to be a perfect _____ (mother, wife, employee, etc.) to be loved/lovable.*
- *I will lose my identity if I'm not the "perfect" person people think I am.*

### Fear-Based Environmental Reactions

Just as you can be reactive to food and other substances (allergies are a good example), your body can have a fear-based reaction to pretty much anything in your environment. This includes foods, substances, people, places, and things. This reaction comes from your body being in a place of fear and defensiveness about something that you come in contact with. I have seen people have negative energetic reactions to their mother, money, a specific color, and more! This reaction just means that your body has decided that that person, place, or thing is dangerous for you. This is very common.

Fearful reactions are an energetic imbalance that can cause almost any "symptom" in the body. Just a few examples include feeling shaky and "off," headaches, itchiness, fatigue, and panic attacks. This is happening because at some point you came into contact with a person, place, or thing *while* you were feeling strong emotion or stress—either related or not related directly to it. Let me explain.

Let's take the example of a family gathering, as this is one I've seen countless times. Everyone is sitting around the coffee table chatting on Thanksgiving when your brother Billy starts ranting about his political views. At the time, you are munching on chocolate-covered almonds, wondering when he will start to attack you about your views, as he always does. As the fear builds, you might have a belief being triggered, such as "I'm unsafe when Billy is unhappy." Or you might recall, subconsciously, an old fight you had with him in the past (an unprocessed experience). During this time, your body is becoming more and more stressed.

While the threat of the family brawl is what's really upsetting to you, your body decides to blame the chocolate-covered almonds you are eating because you are in contact with them at the time. Your energy system then creates a program to "react" to chocolate and almonds so that you are protected from this stress again. Or maybe it doesn't link the chocolate or almonds, but instead it "blames" your brother's unruly dog that is running around the house, so you become reactive to dogs. As another quick example, when we recently got a new kitten in our house, I immediately started feeling fatigued and heavy-headed. After realizing it was a reaction to our fluffy little Stanley, I worked on clearing it. I released fear around responsibility for a new pet and also cleared a couple of unprocessed experiences linked to previous pets. In just a few hours, the symptoms were almost completely gone. If your system perceives that something is a danger to you, it can create this negative reaction in an effort to keep you away from it in the future. It's simply a misdirected protection mechanism.

Your body can become fearful or reactive to anything you are in contact with during times of great stress if the emotional energy doesn't get acknowledged and processed in a healthy way. A lot of these negative reactions will clear as you work on unprocessed experiences and harmful beliefs. However, you can target them directly as well.

## How to Clear Fear

Clearing these types of reactions can be complex, but I'd like to give you a basic technique to use, as it often works quite well. While there is really no clear formula for figuring out what's behind these reactions, a lot of guessing and muscle testing will do the trick.

Using muscle testing, ask: "Is _____ (person, place, or thing) causing a negative reaction in my body?" Then, as we have done before, use muscle testing to ask if you need to know more before you can clear the negative reaction.

If you get a "yes," you will likely need to handle it one of the following ways:

- Find and clear an unprocessed experience linked to it using Thymus Test and Tap and/or EFT.
- Find a harmful belief caused by fear, such as "almonds are dangerous for me," and clear it using Chakra Tapping.

If you get a "no," it means you don't need to know more about why the reaction is happening before you can successfully clear the reaction. You can use this quickie EFT tapping script that I use very successfully to clear fear-based reactions. You can alter the words as long as you are addressing the same theme: the body not liking, being defensive around, and feeling unsafe with the substance or issue you are reacting to. If the item you are reacting to is something tangible (like a type of food or fabric), it's helpful to put it on your lap while you use this script.

**Karate chop point**—*Even though I have this reaction to* _____, *I choose to change that pattern.* Repeat this three times while tapping the karate chop point continuously.

*Rest of the points:*

**Top of the head**—*My body doesn't like* _____.

**Eyebrow**—*My body is really scared of* _____.

**Side of the eye**—*For some reason, my body doesn't like*_____.

**Under the eye**—*I am so defensive around* _____.

**Under the nose**—*My body got the idea that this is scary!*

**Chin**—*This* _____ *is dangerous for me.*

**Collarbone**—*My body can't handle* _____.

**Under the arm/side of body**—*This strong reaction to* _____.

**Top of the hand**—Do the following as you continue to tap:
Close your eyes, open your eyes, shift your eyes down and to the right (don't move your head), shift your eyes down and to the

left (don't move your head), roll your eyes in a big circle in front of you, then roll them in the other direction, hum a few seconds of a song (anything will do!), count to five quickly out loud (1, 2, 3, 4, 5), then hum for a few more seconds.

**Fingertips**—*My body doesn't like _____.*

*My body is really scared of _____.*

*For some reason, my body doesn't like _____.*

*I'm ready to be friends with _____ now.*

*I can be perfectly okay with _____.*

**Back to karate chop**—*My body can relax around _____ now.* (It's beneficial to continue tapping the karate chop point continuously while repeating this one a few times.)

It's good to repeat this process for a few full rounds.

When you've done your clearing, it's important to see if it's really clear. The best way to confirm that your work is done is to muscle-test again. I typically use the testing statement *This _____ is 100 percent safe for me now.* Once you get a "yes" response from the body, the person, place, or thing should no longer cause a negative reaction for you. If possible, it's beneficial to wait twenty-four hours before coming in contact with that reactive energy again.

In addition, the next time you come in contact with that reactive energy, I suggest that you use your EFT tapping points to tap for about one minute before and after contact. You do not need to say anything; rather, just tap the points while in the presence of that energy in order to help reinforce the calm and balanced state. This only needs to be done with the first contact after clearing.

You can also use the EFT tapping points to ease a sudden reaction you are having to something like a food or substance. I've helped many people through swollen tongues, itchy faces, and rashes just by tapping through the points for several rounds (no need to say anything out loud while you tap). The tapping can work wonders to calm down the system, especially while you are determining what medical help you might need, if any.

While I've worked with many clients who have successfully cleared major reactions, I do not recommend you rely solely on this process for anything you are highly reactive to. Allergic reactions are considered a medical issue and can be quite serious, so it's best to be extra cautious.

> *Tip:* You don't need to be scared that you'll create negative environmental fears or reactions every time you're stressed. That's the whole point of all the work we're doing. We're changing our internal relationship with stresses and chaos and more so that our system can better handle things and we can be well.

Through exploring all of these different ways that fear can show up in your life, you are probably now seeing fear in new ways. I've already given you some ideas of unprocessed experiences and beliefs to work with, which will help dissolve fear.

Next, we're going to dig deeper into the process of clearing.

## How to Address Fear Completely

Unprocessed experiences and harmful beliefs are held in the body as a reference point for fear. In other words, experiences and the beliefs that come from them are the body's "proof" that there is something to be scared about, even though the original state of fear may be long past. The beliefs and experiences are essentially "fear triggers." Clearing experiences and beliefs that are acting as fear triggers is one part of clearing fear completely. The body also has a physiological response to fear (the fight, flight, or freeze response), and that can be a very entrenched pattern. It needs to be calmed down, retrained, and redirected to do something different from what it's been doing probably for a very long time. Changing this physiological response to fear is the second part of clearing fear completely. I've seen many "conquer fear" plans fail because one of these aspects was missed. Let me spell out exactly how we achieve fear-clearing success in two parts.

*Part 1: Clear Fear Triggers*

We now know all of the things that can cause fear. Remember, every fear most likely comes down to a core worry that you'll end up unsafe in some way. So if you think in terms of what things make you feel that way, you'll always be on the right track. Clearing those causes are a big part of the overall process of addressing fear. We will do this by using techniques you've already learned to release harmful beliefs and unprocessed experiences.

Here's a breakdown of the process:

- **Clear Unprocessed Experiences**—Identify and clear unprocessed experiences from your past where you may have gone into fight, flight, or freeze mode. This can include experiences where you felt fearful, panicked, humiliated, or unsafe in any way (emotionally or physically). You can jump back to chapter 7 to do this. Additionally, you can use the 3 Hearts Method that you learned in chapter 9. These may include generational or past-life experiences, which we talked about earlier.

- **Clear Harmful Beliefs**—Look at each of the common ways fear can show up, which we just covered. Try to identify harmful beliefs that could be behind them. You can use the suggestions I offered, or you may be able to come up with some of your own. You can go back to chapter 8 to run through that process, or you can use the 3 Hearts Method that you learned in chapter 9. These beliefs may include generational or past-life experiences.

Take your time and gently work on clearing energy using the methods you've learned. Even finding small relief from one fear can help catapult your body in the direction of healing. Go where your heart tells you to go and you'll be moving further away from fear with every step.

*Part 2: Reprogram the Fear Response in the Body*

While it's important to go back and clear the root causes of fear energy, you also need to retrain the fight, flight or freeze response in the body.

Here I'll share several ways to approach this so you can find what works best for you. Remember that we can manipulate and calm that triple warmer meridian (papa bear) energy, which is closely connected to the fear response. By doing so over and over, we can set a new pattern.

By using these simple techniques anytime you're feeling fearful, you'll essentially be saying to your body, *Hey, we can do this calming thing instead now.* You don't have to use them all, but I want to give you several options so you find a few that you feel called to use. You must remember to use them, and to use them consistently, when you get triggered into fear mode. That's the only way this reprogramming process will work.

**Heartbeat Thymus Tapping**—We originally discussed the importance of the thymus gland and tapping it in chapter 4. We then explored it further in chapter 7 when we learned Thymus Test and Tap. Gently tapping the thymus gland in a specific 1-2-3 rhythm, to mimic a heartbeat, is one of my favorite go-to fear-calming techniques. It is both stimulating to the immune system and calming to the body. It's a perfect combination.

I use a flat hand against my chest for this, tapping my fingers against my thymus with the third "beat," or tap, slightly firmer than the rest. This can be done for a few seconds to a few minutes.

**Use the Panic Point**—Remember the "top of the hand," or gamut point, that we use in EFT? It's in the groove between the pinky and ring finger, about halfway down on the top of the hand. Simply use three or four fingers of your other hand and tap or rub that spot. Use it along with deep breaths when you need to calm down. This one is easy to do under a restaurant table or a desk. Because it's directly on the triple warmer meridian or energy pathway, working with it actually sends a message to that energy force to calm down and "back off" from being in overprotective mode.

**Nose Breathing**—When we are panicked, we tend to breathe rapidly through our mouths. If you've ever had a panic attack, you will know just what kind of breathing I'm talking about. One of the ways to signal to the body that we are safe is to adjust our breathing to match the natural breathing pattern of actually feeling safe. For this, I recommend concentrating on nose breathing. Take deep, slow breaths, inhaling and exhaling through your nose. Try to inhale over a period of three seconds, then exhale using that same time goal. It is impossible to breathe rapidly using this method, which helps you gently bring your body back to a calm place. Additionally, slowing down your physical movements during activities like eating or walking signals to the nervous system to slow and calm down as well.

**Panic Pose**—Crossing your arms, which mimics holding or hugging yourself, is extremely calming and protecting. In fact, if you cup each hand so it's cradling the elbow of the opposite arm and gently rock, you'll double your panic-releasing superpower. By rocking, you are triggering the calming response familiar to us all at a primal level, from the time we were first rocked as infants.

**EFT or Chakra Tapping**—Without saying anything at all, tapping the Emotional Freedom Technique (EFT) points or the Chakra Tapping points will work to calm your body when you're in a place of fear. The verbiage we used during the tapping processes in chapters 7 and 8 helped us bring up the energy in order to clear it. However, if you are already in a place of fear, there is no need to say anything. Just allow yourself to be where you are, and tap away until the energy shifts. Once you've calmed down, you can then figure out what triggered you (an unprocessed experience?) and go back to work on that.

**Triple Warmer Meridian Trace**—As you first learned in chapter 2, the triple warmer meridian, or that inner "papa bear" energy, is responsible for your fight, flight, or freeze response. When this meridian becomes overcharged, your body is likely to feel full of adrenaline and panic. Luckily, there is a great way to tame this specific meridian. We can do this by tracing the triple warmer meridian backward. This will gently release or draw out any excess energy that is not needed in the moment. It may be helpful to take a quick look back at the triple warmer meridian image in chapter 2 before you start.

Place each of your hands flat against either side of your face, so your fingertips are resting on your temples and your palms are resting on your cheeks. Now slowly and deliberately trace your hands up and around your ears (staying in contact with your head) as if you were pushing a child's hair back out of their face to comfort them while they were upset. Once you've traced to under your earlobes, continue by dragging your flat hands down the sides of your neck until you reach your shoulders. This should all be one fluid movement. Now lift your hands off, cross your arms so each hand is resting on the opposite shoulder, and continue to slide each hand down your arms so you're in a self-hug position, ending when you are holding your own hands. Take a deep breath. Repeat several more times.

**Create a Safe Space**—Having an accessible go-to plan, or a metaphorical safe space, even in the midst of chaos and doubt can make a huge difference. Here are some suggestions for creating that safe space for yourself, no matter where you are.

- **Choose a Phrase or Symbol**—It's a good idea to create a code phrase or symbol to instantly send ourselves a reminder message that we are safe. My favorite affirmations or mantras for this are "I am safe" and "all is well." You can choose anything you want, but be sure you are saying something you believe at some level, even if it's "I can get through this moment." For symbols that bring comfort, assign yourself a calming image to call upon when you are struggling. It can be anything that has only a positive connotation for you—a religious symbol, the beach, or the smiling face of a baby in your life. If you want to "set" this image as your safe place, simply bring the visual to mind and say, "From now on, when I picture this image, it shall bring me peace, calm, and comfort." Now you can bring it to mind anytime and draw its positive energy right into your body and space.

- **Use Music**—Music, because it has its own energetic frequencies, can be very calming and healing. A special type of sound healing therapy called *Solfeggio frequencies* are believed to date back to ancient Gregorian chants and contain special frequencies. Many people who use them have experienced great benefit. However, I believe that any music you resonate with can have immense healing capability.

  Even though I am not religious, I just love church hymns and gospel church music to calm and center me. I listen to them often as a way to raise my vibration. My favorite for shifting my mood is Smokey Robinson's music. When I'm feeling vulnerable or uncertain, I always listen to Sara Bareilles's song "Brave." It changes everything for me. Having a few different songs that you can use to help create a safe space or shift your vibration can be a great tool.

  Once your body is "trained" into relaxation mode using the songs of your choice, the songs can then be used as an instant calming cue to your body.

* * * * * * * *

You now have lots of tools for calming fear. Use them in the moments when you are feeling fear, and over time your body will be trained into feeling calm instead of going into its usual fear response. While I have offered you many options, you might resonate with only a few. It's okay to use the ones you are drawn to over and over in your practice and disregard anything that you don't resonate with.

Next, you're going to learn how to create a unique map for your own healing using everything you've learned. This is going to pull it all together for you so you have a clear plan to move forward with.

# Section *III*

\* \* \* \* \* \* \* \* \* \* \* \* \* \* \*

# Final Insights
# and Encouragement

\* \* \* \* \* \* \* \* \* \* \* \* \*

### Chapter Eleven

# Create Your Unique Map for Healing

*Take the first step in faith. You don't have to see
the whole staircase, just take the first step.*
—MARTIN LUTHER KING JR., *LET NOBODY TURN US AROUND*

You'll recognize this big, beautiful tree (you!) from earlier. Now that
you've learned about each aspect of my approach to healing, I'm offering you this Healing Tree illustration as an awesome tool to streamline
the whole process of healing. This is your map for becoming who you
really are. In this chapter, you will learn how to use this illustration in
conjunction with the techniques you learned in part three. This simple
process will be your new guide.

At the end of this chapter, you will learn how to establish a new
routine using techniques you've already learned, to help anchor all this
great work you are doing.

## Use the Healing Tree Illustration
You now have the knowledge and understanding to do great healing.
By using the Healing Tree illustration, along with muscle testing and
three simple questions, you'll have a new guide map.

If you are not yet confident in your muscle testing, simply look at the
Healing Tree illustration (instead of using the muscle testing laid out in
the following section) and use your gut to guide you. Trust what is calling to you and you can't go wrong.

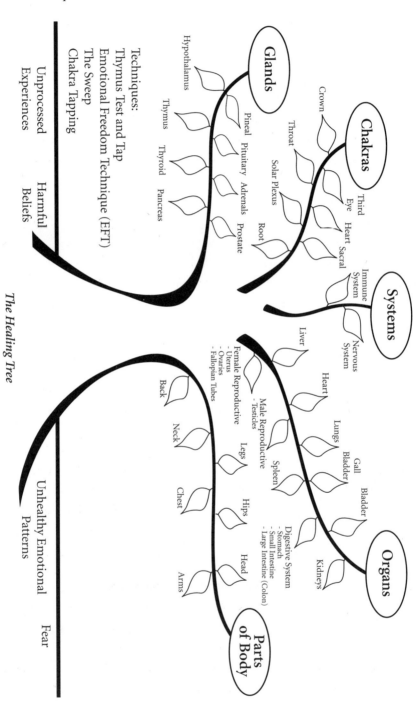

*The Healing Tree*

### Question 1

Ask via muscle testing: "Would it be most beneficial for me to work on _____?"

Fill in the blank with something from either the top section or the soil section of the Healing Tree illustration. Either one is totally fine, but you need to start with one or the other. You'll see why in a minute.

Here are some examples of ways you could start (choose only one):

"Would it be most beneficial for me to work on an organ?" (Top section of the tree.)

If you get a "yes," start asking about organs. Example: "Would it be most beneficial for me to work on my liver?"

"Would it be most beneficial for me to work on my bladder?" (Top section of the tree.)

Did you get a "no?" Okay, then try again.

"Would it be most beneficial for me to work on my liver?" (Top section of the tree.)

OR

"Would it be most beneficial for me to work on a belief?" (Soil section.)

OR

"Would it be most beneficial for me to work on a past experience?" (Soil section.)

OR

"Would it be most beneficial for me to work on a gland?" (Top section of the tree.)

Get the idea here? There isn't any specific order to go in. If you have recurring bladder infections, you might want to just start with your bladder. If you are working on reversing an autoimmune process, you might choose to ask about your immune system first. Thyroid troubles?

Try that first. Panic attacks? Look for fears, harmful beliefs, and unprocessed experiences first. You can refer to chapter 6 for some ideas, too.

Do remember, though, that with any condition or challenge, there are various contributing components of that larger issue. For example, if you want to work on something like low-functioning adrenals, it is likely that there are other imbalances in your body linked to that, perhaps nervous-system stress and low thyroid function, among other things. You'll be most successful if, in addition to working on the larger challenge, you also "think small" and work on a more detailed scale as well. Again, just follow your body's lead. Do you remember the story of my client with digestive issues who lost her fear of speaking on the phone without us ever addressing that fear directly? Let it serve as a reminder that seemingly unrelated-to-your-biggest-challenge things are beneficial to work on, too. Clearing energy linked to anything you see on the Healing Tree illustration will help you move in the right direction. And remember, you won't need to clear it all in order to heal.

Once you have determined where you'll start, you're ready for your next step. You need to get more clues so you can find something specific to work on. Just knowing you want to start with a belief or your bladder isn't quite enough yet. You need more details.

If you started with the *top* section of the tree, you're basically now going to find out what from the *soil* section of the illustration is causing an imbalance in that area of your body.

If you started with the soil section of the illustration, just hang tight. You're set for now.

### Question 2

If you started with the *top* section of the tree illustration, muscle-test this question: "Is there a _____ (insert something from the soil section) causing stress on my bladder?"

When you find out what it is—a belief, an unprocessed experience, fear, or an unhealthy emotional pattern—you just need to ask one more question before you start.

## Question 3

We always have to give the body a chance to let us know why something is an issue. You will remember doing this in previous chapters. Ask and muscle-test this question: "Do I need to know more about this before I clear it?"

If you get a "no," your body is saying it's ready to clear this, pronto. If you get a "yes," just know that this is part of the acknowledgment process your body requires in order to let it go. This will require a bit of detective work. You can basically just ask questions of yourself, like you would to a friend if they had this issue. Just guess what could be connected to the issue.

To get to that information, you can ask questions like this: "Is it linked to _____?" (You can also use the words "connected to," "triggered by," or anything else fitting for you.) Here are some possibilities for how to fill in the blank:

- a person (family member, friend, teacher, colleague, neighbor)
- career
- school
- a place (a certain house, a city, etc.)
- a thing (a food, a car, etc.)

For each clue you come up with, you should repeat that question, if you are using muscle testing: "Do I need to know more about this before I clear it?"

When your body says "no," or you can't come up with any more clues by using your conscious thinking, you're going to head off armed with that information. You can now flip to the appropriate chapter and do the clearing. You may be able to clear all of it at once, or you may have to come back at different times, working slowly as your body is able.

Remember, when you are done, double-check that the issue is clear from your system. Ask something like, "Is _____ still causing stress in my body?"

When you're done, come back to the Healing Tree illustration.
Breathe.
Repeat.

*Tip:* I've mentioned briefly before that if you are comfortable
with muscle testing, I recommend asking your body which of
the five main techniques would be most beneficial to clear with.
As a reminder, the five techniques are: Thymus Test and Tap,
Emotional Freedom Technique, The Sweep, Chakra Tapping,
and the 3 Hearts Method.

To figure out which technique will work best, you can ask, "Would
it be most beneficial to clear this _____ (insert issue) with _____
(insert technique)?" Keep guessing until you get a "yes."

You may need to layer techniques to gently clear the energy, so be
open to coming back and asking that question again if necessary. You
can tweak the technique to fit your specific situation and explore what
works for you, and when. That's exactly how I developed my own effective protocols. I just kept trying new things and revising.

## A Healing Tree Example

Here's how using the concept of the Healing Tree illustration supported me in helping a client with severe and persistent migraines.

When Janet first came to me, she had no idea what was triggering
recent headaches. Janet was a high-powered executive, and while the
headaches were a new symptom, her stress levels were long-standing. I
thought of some clues her body could be offering (from chapter 6). We
identified that she was constantly "doing her head in" wondering what
other people thought of her. Even though she ran this huge company,
she still worried incessantly about judgment from clients and even her
own employees.

Working with that plausible idea, I intuitively chose an element of
the Healing Tree illustration to start with. I often use muscle testing, but
my intuition sometimes takes over and I just go in that direction first.
Never be afraid to use your intuition, as it will become more accurate as
you become better attuned to your body. I thought it was probably an

unprocessed experience (from the soil section of the illustration) and then muscle-tested it for confirmation: "Are the headaches linked to an unprocessed experience?" (If you don't have any idea of which one to choose first, just guess one by one). Her body responded with a "yes." So we set off to find the experience. We asked if the experience was linked to a specific age. We got a "no." Then we asked if the experience was linked to a specific person. We got a "yes." After more guessing and muscle testing, we traced the experience back to a teacher she'd had in both first and second grade. The teacher had made her go in front of the class to read a story she wrote and then asked the other kids to give the story a grade. Janet still cringed when she thought about this. We now had an unprocessed experience to work with. We cleared that using Thymus Test and Tap and Emotional Freedom Technique, and then just kept going—asking and clearing.

## Additional Questions to Unlock Your Healing

As you practice the concepts and techniques you've learned in this book, you will become more relaxed and less methodical. You will see there is a very organic unfolding to all of this, and it needs no organization or order. All roads lead you to healing. Your intuition will kick in more often, and you may not need to use the Healing Tree illustration every time. Things will pop into your head (this is often your subconscious pushing forward ideas for you), and you'll have more of your own leads to follow. You might use some of the following questions to ignite your intuition. In time, you will find you have your own set of questions that help you get just the answers you need for your healing.

- "Do I have a belief causing stress on my immune system?" You can substitute "immune system" with "adrenal glands," "nervous system," etc.
- "Do I have a belief causing dysfunction in my _____ (name an organ, muscle, or gland of your choice)?"
- "Is there an experience from my past that is making it difficult for me to heal?"

- "Is there an unhealthy relationship in my life causing stress on my body?" Note: It's important to know that while a person in your life may seem like the problem, it's most likely your reaction to that person that is causing the problem for you. For example, the fact that your brother refuses to listen to you about how to raise his kids does not mean your brother is a problem. The real issue causing distress is your reaction to your brother. You can clear beliefs, unprocessed experiences, and fear patterns triggered by certain people with the various techniques you already know.

- "Do I have a belief that makes me feel I need this _____ (state the illness, problem, or challenge)?"

- "Is my difficulty healing linked to a specific negative emotional pattern?" Ask about each pattern we covered, individually.

- "Is my _____ (state the organ, muscle, gland, or part of the body that is manifesting symptoms) trying to give me a message?"

- "Is there a specific experience that my body is storing that is keeping me in fight, flight, or freeze mode?"

- "Do I need to forgive myself for something from my past in order to heal?"

- "Is there a benefit to this _____ (state the illness, problem, or challenge) that is making it difficult for me to heal?"

- "Is there an experience I need to heal in order to raise my body's vibration?"

- "Is there a frequency in my body that is a match for _____ (parasites, viruses, bacteria, etc.)?" Note: This question fits in with the concept of the law of attraction. Releasing any emotional energy that is an energetic match to the parasite, virus, bacteria, etc., will help you to heal from it.

- "Am I holding generational energy that is having a negative impact on my body?"

- "Am I holding past-life energy that is having a negative impact on my body?"
- "Would it be beneficial to release energy related to _____?" Here are some possibilities for how you could fill in the blank:
  - a person (family member, friend, teacher, colleague, neighbor)
  - career
  - school
  - a place (a certain house you lived in, a city, or anything else you can think of)
  - a thing (a food, a car, etc.)

Between using the Healing Tree illustration process, the additional suggested questions I've offered, and your own developing intuition, you have a plethora of ideas to work with. Now it's time to learn how to encourage a new positive pattern in your body.

## Create a New Routine

You now know that a huge part of healing is about releasing negative energy from our systems. As we make a dent in that work, we are slowly building ourselves back up in the way we were intended to be. Creating a routine in order to help establish a positive pattern is just as important as clearing a negative one.

Routine has never been a strong point of mine. I'm more of a fly-by-the-seat-of-my-flowy-skirt kind of girl. But I've learned that setting up some routine practices can be hugely beneficial in helping us stay on the right track. Just as I've always found it easier to maintain my weight than to gain weight and have to lose it later, I've had a similar experience with healing. It's far easier for me to keep on top of this energy-balancing business than to allow myself to slip backward and end up with a big pile of stuff to dig through again.

I've learned this lesson more times than I can count—on both hands. It goes like this. I'm on a roll. I feel good. I get busy. I think I don't need to do anything to remain in this flow of awesomeness. But then, little by little, I start to ignore small things, I overwork instead of allow myself the time I need, I skip doing things that are important to me, and so it goes. I start to feel a little rickety, and then a little more. Eventually, I always end up thinking, *Wow, that would have been way less annoying if I'd just done what I knew I needed to do in the first place.* Now, this doesn't mean I've been perfect at this even with these reminders, and it's unlikely you will be either. That's completely okay. Life is about sometimes slipping up, staying up too late, reminding ourselves that we're not completely invincible, and having too much fun, chocolate, and wine. This certainly doesn't hurt unless it becomes the new routine. Don't beat yourself up. Just say, "Oh, there it is again. This is very human!" Then start again.

If you have some of your own practices, like yoga, meditation, or deep breathing, then consider using them along with any bits and pieces of techniques you've learned in this book. These will ideally be simple things instead of, say, the entire version of a clearing technique. Many things can even be done in the shower, so there's really no excuse not to drop them into your schedule. When you're just sitting watching TV, see if you can work one in. During a bathroom break, take an extra few minutes to do something calming or healing. This doesn't have to feel like a big chore or project. Your only mistake is doing nothing at all. You can do some of these before you get out of bed in the morning.

I'm all about integrating these techniques into your life instead of adding them to your to-do list. You can find a few practices and do them all together as a morning ritual, turn them into a before-bed routine, or scatter them throughout your day.

Here are a few suggestions of techniques to integrate into your day:

- Grounding
- Tracing around the eyes

- Thymus tapping
- Tapping through the Emotional Freedom Technique (EFT) points
- A few minutes of chanting

It doesn't matter what your new routine consists of; it just matters that you create one that feels good to your body. This practice of creating healthy energy patterns by using a routine is like a retraining process for your body. It will return rewards far bigger than the effort.

*Chapter Twelve*

\* \* \* \* \* \* \* \* \* \* \* \* \* \* \*

# Keep Moving Forward

*When nothing seems to help, I go back and look at the stonecutter hammering away at his rock, perhaps a hundred times without as much as a crack showing in it. Yet at the hundred and first blow it will split in two, and I know it was not that blow that did it—but all that had gone before.*

—JACOB RIIS

While my own healing journey felt erratic, with many ups and downs and in-betweens, each person's will be different. And however yours plays out, it's quite all right. There will be times that feel like smooth sailing, and others that feel like the healing seas are so tumultuous, you could be seasick. It's all part of your ultimate healing.

It is often impossible to tell what's going on inside of your body during the healing process, and it's easy to feel like nothing is happening at all. I half-laugh, half-cringe now as I remember all of the moments when I would have traded my life savings to get one sneak peek into that body and brain of mine. I so often felt like I was looking into a clouded fishbowl trying to get a glimpse into one clear space of me to decipher what the heck was going on. And sometimes you will be that fishbowl, too.

As you move through those moments, being aware of patterns and receiving insight into what might be happening can be immensely helpful. I'm going to outline those patterns for you here.

## Healing Patterns

While we need to learn to be okay with not always being able to constantly monitor our progress, there are some common healing patterns that I've seen over the years that will give you a little bit of inspiration to keep on keepin' on. You may recognize one of these, or all of them, as your own. Our patterns of healing can be not only very different from each other but also different for us at different times in our own lives. Remember, by the time your body reaches the point of manifesting physical symptoms, the energetic imbalances have already been there for some time. The same idea applies to the manifestation of physical healing. The repair work often goes on for a long time before your body reaches the point of physical changes. There are many people who say that they suddenly, miraculously, healed. While healing can *seem* sudden, it's usually not. It's just that the culmination of all that has been happening appears at once.

I liken the process of healing to the growth of a baby. Imagine that a pregnant mother, desperate to see her growing baby, demands that her doctor perform a daily ultrasound as proof of the baby's progress. It would be impossible to see the tiny day-to-day changes occurring in the baby's growth, but at the end of nine months, the baby will have legs and arms and internal organs. Your healing is happening like this for you, too. It's often impossible to see or feel these tiniest of shifts, but that doesn't mean they aren't happening.

You *are* healing. It *is* happening—even if you can't see it quite yet.

### Pattern A: Ups, (Melt) Downs, and In-Betweens

There is one clue you can bet your money on that indicates you're most definitely healing. It's feeling an improvement in your *emotional* state of being. It can be even just 1 percent. Feeling better, or sturdier, emotionally is rock-solid evidence that you are well on your way to more improvements. The key is to allow that to be enough until the physical manifestations show up.

As you move along your healing journey, you will have moments or maybe even minutes or days when you feel like you are returning to yourself or your symptoms are waning. You will have a deep sense of all being well, knowing you will somehow, inevitably, be okay. This feeling may be fleeting, lasting only seconds at first, but you'll recognize it. This is a glimpse of what is to come and stay. You may get the glimpses only occasionally at first, but over time they will occur closer together or perhaps last a bit longer. One day you will realize that although you still have many subpar moments to count, it is as if someone is stitching together the glimpses for you into the picture of health you want. If you can enjoy the glimpses while they are present, forming no attachment to holding on to them for fear they will leave, I promise they will return. Just think of them as your angels saying, "Keep going. You're on the right track. We're helping to make this a full-time gig for you."

As an example, I'll share a story about a client I worked with for a few months. Cindy was dealing with fibromyalgia. At the beginning of each session when I would call her, I would have no idea what kind of report I would get. It seemed like things were all over the place for her. She would be feeling stable one day, and then the next day it would feel to her as if the world were crashing down. Then she'd get over the hump and return to her baseline again (which was not, by the way, feeling good). But we kept on keeping on, knowing the work would be fruitful.

One day when we were talking during a session, she said, "Amy, I had this really weird experience. I was walking the dog the other day, and for a few minutes, it was like all was right in the world. I had this deep sense of peace and wellness. Then I lost it."

"Great!" I exclaimed. "You got your first glimpse of what's on its way to you." Cindy then went back to the same pattern of what had been happening prior to this, for quite some time. And then she got another glimpse. Eventually, she was getting glimpses more often and they were starting to be only days apart from each other. Eventually, but not without experiencing more meltdowns, her body started to "hold" or be in alignment with these glimpses more and more. In just another few months, her reference point for her own stability had kicked up a few notches. Her "new normal" was a much better-feeling normal than it had been in the past, and the glimpses kept coming. When we stopped working together, it was because Cindy knew she only had to keep moving forward in the way we had been together. Her good days now outnumbered her bad. And the meltdowns? They still show up sometimes, but she works through them, imagining that each one allows space in her experience for another, or longer, "glimpse."

It is so very common to be moving forward and then suddenly feel like you are back at a low again, continuing in this pattern during the entire healing process until the next dip happens. Actually, doesn't life sometimes go like this, too? This is the healing pattern that most people resonate with, though: up, meltdown, up, meltdown, and so on—but eventually the "up" holds. Hitting a low does not in any way mean that you are starting over. Healing can be just like climbing to a peak. It's likely that you will stumble at times as you climb, but you will get back up and continue on. Great things await.

### Pattern B: Physical and Emotional Retracing

Retracing is a concept that I really started to come to understand, although somewhat hesitantly, during my time in India. Chiropractic, homeopathic, and naturopathic practitioners recognize and acknowledge this concept, but Western medical practitioners rarely do. Some people say this is because mainstream medical approaches rarely produce retracing reactions.

The retracing process is essentially one of a disease reversing itself—and it's not always fun. It consists of retracing time periods from the past (and the symptoms that went with it) until the individual reaches the point from which they started.

While healing, it's possible that you will "retrace" or experience symptoms that have not been present for months or even years. This can be so confusing, and can leave you feeling like you are getting worse or developing some new problem. But often these symptoms are actually a process of retracing the several stages through which the disease manifested. To many doctors and practitioners, these retracing symptoms are a positive indication that the body is healing and returning to normal function.

Old injuries can "turn on" or flare again and then simply go away. Emotional states will do the same: turn on, run their course, and then simply disappear. Retracing symptoms can be related to eliminating toxic substances, healing chronic infections, healing old emotional traumas, energetic imbalances, or simply metabolic shifts that take place as a body heals and its vitality increases. Retracing symptoms can last days or weeks, though usually not more than that.

It's very difficult to identify retracing, but I've found a few markers:

- Were you starting to feel better before the "crash"? When the body has more energy, it is more likely to initiate a retracing process.

- Have the symptoms occurred in the past without returning for a long time but are now popping up again? These "surprise symptoms" often come back for a last round of deep healing.

- Is your protocol one that rebalances the energy or chemistry of the body at a holistic level? As the body's balance improves, old memories and toxicity often surface to be released.

Long before my Lyme diagnosis, I went to a neurologist who discovered that my myelin sheaths—the outer coverings of the nerves—were degenerating at a rapid pace. I was put on a therapy called IVIG, which stands for intravenous immune globulin. IVIG is a solution of concentrated antibodies extracted from healthy donors, which the recipient gets via infusion to treat disorders of the immune system or to boost immune response. During this treatment, the nearly intolerable nerve pain I was experiencing was severely heightened. My neurologist assured me that sometimes regenerating can be as or more painful than degenerating. He explained that even though the nerves were being repaired, they were being stimulated and agitated just as much as during the degeneration process. And over time, I did definitely feel like the IVIG helped, despite the feeling at the time that it was making things worse.

During my adventures in healing my menstrual issues, I recognized the same pattern. I think that my body, finally having had several good months, was strong enough to go back and heal some old, deep imbalances.

Retracing is a common part of healing, but you also want to make sure something new is not developing. Only a medical professional can determine this. Always check with your doctor or practitioner if a new symptom arises.

### Pattern C: Baby Steps

This is the "slow and steady wins the race" kind of pattern. It's the pattern where the person slowly improves over time, always moving in a forward direction toward health. They don't deal with consistent setbacks; they simply keep chugging along in the right direction. This was certainly not my own healing pattern for most of my journey, although it tends to show up more in the "home stretch." I'd be lucky if, for a day or two, I wasn't confused about five different possible scenarios or explanations for my bodily chaos. But there are luckier ducks than me.

For example, I started working with Alice after the worst of her Lyme disease experience had passed, but she was far from feeling well or being able to function as she wished. She was still taking several naps a day, was unable to work more than a few hours at a time, and couldn't take the family vacations she desperately desired. During our initial session we cleared three harmful beliefs, a process you learned about in chapter 8. From that day, Alice was on a baby-steps path to complete wellness. Slowly but surely, with very few major meltdowns or setbacks, she continued to improve. Within a month, she was able to naturally wean herself from naps. Within several more months, she was able to work an entire day doing the job she loved. And the first summer after we started working together, she joined her family for a hiking trip and out-hiked a few of the avid athletes! She simply needed a kick-start, and releasing those initial energetic blocks definitely did the trick.

## Ease Discomfort During Processing

During and after energy work, remember that you are shifting and rebalancing. You might remember from earlier that we call this time period *processing*. Your body and its energy "field," which extends far beyond your actual physical being, are simply going through an adjustment process. Not everyone feels these shifts as discomfort, or at all. However, if you should, here are a few things that will help ease the process:

- Drink extra water, as being dehydrated will make it difficult for your body's energies to adjust.
- Take a break for a day or so from doing big clearings until your body catches up.
- Use Emotional Freedom Technique or Chakra Tapping along with the following script:

  Karate chop point: *Even though I feel worse right now, I choose to let this energy move through me.*

  *Even though I feel* _____ *(explain how you feel), I can let my body rebalance now.*

  *Even though I'm not feeling good, I can be okay.*

  Then on the rest of the points, whether you are using EFT or Chakra Tapping, tap through and just vent about how you feel. When you are ready to wrap up, do one final round on all the points, focusing on some simple positive statements, such as *I can be okay, All is well now*, or any other phrases that are comforting to you.

- Do some grounding (from chapter 4).

These practices should help get you through any rough spots and keep you moving along in a forward direction.

## Helpful Reminders

I remember the days when people would say to me, "I just don't know how you do it, Amy." I always explained, "I wake up every day and it's there to do." And so it is. You just keep going. You keep waking up. You learn more and ultimately, with each sunrise, you find ways to make the doing not so scary.

Eventually you might realize you've been doing and surviving for a long while, more than you ever thought you could. The fact that you're still waking up, and finding new days to try new ways of living, says you're pretty darn good at it. When you start to see that, you'll feel better and better. You'll start to slowly sneak away from the struggle until one day you'll wake up and, without even trying, it won't be *so hard* anymore. You won't be doing it. You'll have done it!

Because I know what it's like when feeling good seems to be light-years away, I want you to have insights to help you be more comfortable as you go through the process. You're setting a new and healthier pattern, one that keeps on saying to your body through redirection of the energy, "*This* way is better." So practice the techniques you've learned throughout the book, wake up each morning, rinse, and repeat. Hopefully these final insights will provide an extra boost for you along the way.

### Learn to Trust

Don't get attached to how healing "should be" or get judgmental about the process. Our "should-be's" create far more emotional and physical stress than the actual event that we're "should-be-ing" about. You are where you are and that's it. It's happening how it's happening and that's that. Try to relax into how it's all unfolding and I promise you'll be where you want to be a whole lot faster.

Each thing you experience—in every minute, hour, and day—whether it appears to be for your benefit or against it, is part of a larger picture. It's all necessary. See it as just that. Stop weighing how much it's worth and just trust that in some way it's necessary for your path simply because it is happening—even through lots of twists and turns that make it look like your goal is lost.

There is a reason for everything that happens in your life: it's getting you somewhere good, it's getting you away from something not so good, or it's happening because it needs to get your attention. Trust that the universe is talking to you and trying to sidestep you into exactly where you need to be. It's all part of the game.

During a trip to India that I took in 2009, two years after my initial trip for stem cells, something happened that was greater than anything I could have ever plotted myself. The night before my plane was to leave for home, I had terrible food poisoning (they call it "Delhi belly"). Hang on, we haven't gotten to the incredible part yet! I was vomiting into a plastic bag, desperate for the comforts of home, yet I knew there was no way I could get on a flight. I called the airline in desperation, and they agreed to reschedule my flight with no penalty or fee.

Days later as I recovered at the hospital, a girl named Charlotte came to visit her mother, who was also a patient at the hospital. My eyes met Charlotte's across the physical therapy room, and in a total plot twist, we fell in love.

Years after that, when my symptoms started to flood back during that trip to London, I was forced to muddle my way through the painful process of healing, having believed illness was already far behind me. This time, though, I had no doctors to rely on. I had to rely on me. And through it, I found myself, and this beautiful work that I get to share with so many people every single day. I have been happier and healthier than ever before.

In 2007 when I made the difficult decision to go to India for stem cells, I never imagined that India would turn out to be such an important part of a bigger picture—part of me meeting my now-wife and of me turning inward for my ultimate healing. I've seen now, countless times, that things often fall apart so they can piece themselves back together again, but in a better way—a universal upgrade of sorts.

### Be Open to a Change in Your Story

This is so important that I almost want to scream it at you! It's easy to keep telling ourselves the same old story: *I don't feel good. I still have so much fear. I'm crying all the time. My body hurts.* But noticing your healing improvements requires eyes that are looking for them. Make sure your eyes are open.

Healing can show up in subtle ways and may look like one of these examples:

- You had a physical or emotional meltdown, but you bounced back even slightly better or faster than the last time.

- After you went out to do something fun, you didn't crash for two days, but just one instead.

- You normally hold on to anger for a long time when someone hurts you. This time when you got hurt, you got just as mad, but you let it go sooner than usual.

- You get tired so easily, but now you walk with a little more pep in your step before totally crashing.

- You get just as tired, but you don't beat yourself up about it as much.

- You just stopped and rested. (A huge sign of emotional healing is being easier on yourself, which then helps to free up energy for physical healing.)

### *Give Yourself Permission to Find What Works for You*

A journal entry from two days before my trip to India in 2007 read: *I hereby vow to heal in every way I can during this trip. I will stretch my healing boundaries and try whatever comes my way. Even the weird shit.*

My kick-start eventually arrived on its own when Dr. Shroff announced she had hired a yogi to teach classes in the hospital's physical therapy room. Everyone I knew who did yoga looooved it. The class was to be held three times a week, free to patients and their families.

Our teacher, Rohit, was easy to read instantly. He was all about the practice and absolutely no fun. Week after week, he directed us to perform our first impossible move and expected nothing less from me than to at least "try, try!" when I insisted aloud that I don't bend that way. "Keep working on your breath. Breeeeaaath makes miracles," he said repeatedly.

I wished I was in love with yoga. I desperately wanted to be one of those students who felt transformed on the mat, wouldn't miss a class, and made my master proud. I was determined to allow myself to quit only after I found the joy everyone else seemed to have in this practice. One day, when Rohit finally stopped reminding me about my form and breathing, I realized I had succeeded. At the end of each session, he always proclaimed, "You are now light and free!" And surprisingly, after hearing him bark for an entire hour in his weighty Indian accent that day, I kinda did feel that way. But during the next class, I was back to dreaming of wandering the city and counting sweat droplets that were falling from my head. That's when I decided that it was my time to exit yogaland gracefully.

Life, like yoga, is all about being okay with exactly where you are. Based on those parameters, I decided I had mastered enough of this practice. I ducked out when the class was over, proud and calm, but mostly relieved that for rest of my trip I could breathe any damn way I wanted. Yoga is amazing, I know. Rohit was dedicated and surely would have helped me become a more limber and disciplined person. But yoga is not for me. And when I became okay with that, I moved on to things that catapulted me further toward health.

Falling into a similar internal-pressure trap when I was first learning about energy therapy, I read a ridiculous number of books on energy therapy, emotional trauma, and mind-body-spirit healing. I studied every program and consumed all of the information I could find on the subjects. What I realized at some point, exhausted by that approach, was that we don't always need *more:* more knowledge, more training, more searching. We just need to find what feels good to us and be with it.

If you resonate deeply with three techniques out of all of them in this book, you have enough to work with. If you resonate with only one technique, you have enough. You'll find a way to use it for everything and be successful. It's not about the quantity; it's about the connection.

Never follow a path, stick with a plan, or convince yourself to agree with anything unless your soul is giving you an affirmative nod. Your healing path will be a unique one, so while you're on your search, be open to everything, but only throw your energy into something that resonates—and know there is a deeper reason you're diggin' it. Or not.

### Maintain a Balanced Focus

There is a learned balance that will come, in time, between making your healing important and making it your entire all-consuming focus.

Just because you know a new technique or approach and have tapped into your own power doesn't mean this should become your life (even though I totally understand the temptation). The concept of "too much of a good thing" is true here for a couple of solid reasons.

First, with energy work, as we briefly touched on earlier, there is a processing that happens as that energy moves out of our field. Until that happens, we might not feel the full shift or improvement. This is similar to how eating doesn't always provide instant fullness. If you just keep eating without seeing how it all settles, you'll do much more harm than good. I can't emphasize enough the importance of giving your body time and space to allow the healing process to happen. Remember, you are trying to create a solution, not more problems— which is precisely what you will do if you push yourself too hard.

Next, focusing too much on something you *don't* want isn't helpful, which we learned in chapter 4 in regard to the law of attraction. While being active in your healing is beneficial, making your whole life *about* your healing is absolutely not. Your world (activities, entertainment, and people) must consist of more than this one goal or focus.

Everyone will have a different way of shifting their focus to achieve this balance. I personally did this in a few different ways. I sometimes drank wine even while knowing green juice would surely be healthier. I watched *Golden Girls* marathons and B-rated movies for hours on end when I could have been meditating. I ate fettuccine Alfredo on occasion, even though I knew dairy could increase inflammation in my body. I did things just for pure pleasure or fun, because pleasure and fun are healing. What I'm saying here is really this: Don't limit your reading list to only books about healing; keep the mindless summer reads, too. Don't be terrified of one bite of sugar. Don't cut yourself off from the reality of life and bury yourself further into a world you are trying to separate from. Because in the big picture, it just doesn't make you or break you. In the big picture, giving yourself more no's does one thing and one thing only: it creates a focus on what you don't have. And absolutely no healing comes from that.

There, I let you off the hook. Integrate these practices you've learned into your life. Embrace them fully, but don't over-focus and exhaust yourself. Find that balance.

### Seek Support

Sometimes the journey can be lonely. We just want someone to understand, cry with us, or shake us out of our current rut. Sometimes we just need help getting to the next step. There is a good reason to ask for help, from either a friend or a professional, and it's not because self-healing doesn't work. It may be true that you *can* heal yourself, but everything is easier when we have a little tribe to help us. You do need to be responsible for your own journey, but you don't have to do it alone.

If you are not working with a professional regularly, check in with yourself to see if it might be beneficial to work with one, at least occasionally. Here's why. A professional has seen hundreds and hundreds of clients, and you've only had experience with, well, you. People who do this all day long have seen different patterns and issues emerge, which gives them an advantage—they can often quickly see what you can't. Not only that, but this is an amazing way to learn how and what to apply for yourself. You will get to see how a professional unravels issues and what they do when they get stuck. You may even hear a story from their own journey that will generate new ideas for your healing.

I regularly have clients who "graduate" from working with me regularly in one-on-one sessions and then contact me for a check-in appointment here and there. They fill me in on what's going on and share any stumbling blocks. From there, I'm always able to give them new ideas or direction they can take on their own for more healing and clearing. This gives them a great new jumping-off point and a little reassurance when they need some confirmation that they are doing just fine. Giving your power away and asking for support are two totally different things. Seeking insight, advice, ideas, and a boost will often allow you to take your healing to the next level.

If you are unable to work with a professional or are uncomfortable doing so, find someone who will help you raise your vibration and help you focus on solutions to feeling better right now. Do not ask for help from those who are struggling too much themselves and are likely to have "contagious panic energy." If you don't have the tribe you desire, you may need to get creative. Find people who lift you up. If you don't have a strong support system in family and friends, look elsewhere. It doesn't take hours of phone time; sometimes just a familiar face and a smile from a neighbor or grocery clerk can truly make a difference.

Always know, too, that you have support from angels, relatives on the other side, and more. You simply need to ask for their help. So often I would, and still do to this day, call out and ask for help from my invisible tribe. You might laugh if you are new to this idea, but they always come through.

Your support system is anyone or anything that makes you feel sturdier and surrounded with comfort. There are opportunities all around. It's your new job to seek them out.

## My Final Note to You

I am not good with endings or goodbyes. I never love writing the last sentence of a book. It often feels sad to part with it all, and by that point, I always wonder, what more of importance can I say that I haven't already said? But there's still something left here—words that I want you to remember in every part of your being.

This is the beginning.

Now is your time. Through this work, you get to experience who you really are and unbury yourself from who you thought you should be.

You get to—possibly for the first time—notice who you are separate from fear, this challenge, this illness. You get to discover your true purpose, which is not at all what you thought it was before. When I was at my sickest in India, Dr. Shroff said to me, "You need to find a purpose. You will heal when you find a purpose. You will heal when you follow your heart." While I didn't understand this at the time, and was convinced my heart had no idea where to lead me anyway, I later came to see exactly what she meant. She wanted me to have something so important to me that I would move beyond what kept me "living small." It wasn't necessarily the passion or the purpose that was important, but more so the distraction from worrying that I wasn't good enough. Because I had work to do. I had places to go. I had people to meet. I had my light to shine. Dr. Shroff wanted me to connect with myself on a deeper level, and having a purpose makes you do that. However, in my delicate state, I amassed an army of internal pressure against myself, adding to my chore list: Find purpose.

I wish someone had said *this* to me at that moment:

When you finally realize that your purpose, and your natural-born right, is only to be happy with who you really are—whether you are a healer or a comedian or someone who smiles at strangers—you trigger a process inside of yourself that is infinitely bigger than whatever is standing in your way at this moment. Happiness is your purpose. And you will come to see, at the end of all your exhaustive searching, that your purpose has never been external. It has not been to make sure others are happy with you. It has not been to be perfect. It has been, from your first day here, to simply allow your expression without thought or hindrance. It doesn't matter where you start, because from that place of whoever you are at the core, you will naturally expand outward into any other secondary missions you may have in this lifetime. Everything is channeled through that first insanely important purpose, which is to find yourself and stay there. It's the spark, the impetus, that sets everything else in motion.

While we have covered massive ground in this book, all that you have learned can be boiled down to a few things that make up the formula for true healing.

You must...

- become who you really are.
- learn to be easy on yourself, and love yourself.
- trust that you can be okay, no matter what.

This may seem overly simplified, but these things will do for you what nothing else can. These are the things that will help you heal in the deepest spaces of your being.

Whether you have read this book and believe you have the power to heal, or you have read this book and aren't quite sure yet, it's okay. Healing takes courage and grace and a sharp turn in the direction away from so much of what you know. But it also takes a fair share of messy, crying-on-the-floor drowning in doubt. During these days, know that you are doing some of your biggest work, too. You are doing what you should have been doing all along. You are doing *you*. You are acting from your true authenticity, free from the filtering or stifling that you came to learn somewhere along the way. Haruki Murakami, in his book *Kafka on the Shore,* wrote: "And once the storm is over, you won't remember how you made it through, how you managed to survive. You won't even be sure, in fact, whether the storm is really over. But one thing is certain. When you come out of the storm, you won't be the same person who walked in. That's what this storm's all about."

Just as it takes a village to raise a child, it takes a whole lotta love to heal. The real truth, though, is that the only love you really need is yours. Healing is sometimes difficult and scary, but remember, you were born brave. You are ready.

# Book Club Discussion Questions

1. What are your greatest fears around healing?

2. If you could frame your healing journey as a book, what would the title be?

3. What was your aha moment in the book? Why?

4. Is there anything you disagree with or don't resonate with from the book? Why?

5. What quotes or lines from the book do you want as a sticky note by your desk or bed?

6. Did this book change your perspective on healing or just confirm what you already believe or know?

7. What parts of the book have you found yourself thinking about the most?

8. Which techniques help you feel the most empowered? Why?

9. Which techniques do you think you're unlikely to use? Why?

10. What's your one big takeaway from the book?

11. Whom do you wish would read this book that you know won't? Why don't you think they would and why do you think they should?

12. How would you describe the book to a friend if you had only a minute (an elevator pitch)?

13. Which parts or techniques are you most likely to share or teach to a loved one? Whom do you most want to share with, and why?

14. How will this book change your future thinking/healing/growth? What will you never look at the same?

15. What part of your healing journey is most confusing or frustrating for you? Is there a technique in the book that could be used to help you move past it? What advice would you give a friend about it in order to help them move forward in their own healing journey?

16. What unhealthy emotional pattern from the book do you feel is most important for you to work on? Is it something you knew before you read the book?

17. If you could ask Amy one question, what would it be?

18. If you'd read this book earlier, do you think it would have changed your path?

* * * * * * * * * * * * * * * *

# Additional Resources

### Books

Brockman, Howard, LCSW. *Dynamic Energetic Healing: Integrating Core Shamanic Practices with Energy Psychology Applications and Processwork Principles.* Columbia Press, 2006.

Dillard, Sherrie. *Develop Your Medical Intuition: Activate Your Natural Wisdom for Optimum Health and Well-Being.* Woodbury, MN: Llewellyn Publications, 2015.

Eden, Donna, with David Feinstein, PhD. *Energy Medicine: Balancing Your Body's Energies for Optimal Health, Joy, and Vitality.* New York: Jeremy P. Tarcher/Putnam, 1998.

Emoto, Masaru. *The Hidden Messages in Water.* New York: Atria Books, 2005.

Feinstein, David, Donna Eden, and Gary Craig. *The Promise of Energy Psychology: Revolutionary Tools for Dramatic Personal Change.* Jeremy P. Tarcher/Penguin, 2005.

Grout, Pam. *E-Squared: Nine Do-It-Yourself Energy Experiments That Prove Your Thoughts Create Your Reality.* Carlsbad, CA: Hay House Insights, 2013.

Hay, Louise L. *You Can Heal Your Life.* Santa Monica, CA: Hay House, 1984.

Hicks, Esther and Jerry. *The Law of Attraction: The Basics of the Teachings of Abraham.* Carlsbad, CA: Hay House, 2006.

Lipton, Bruce H., PhD. *The Biology of Belief: Unleashing the Power of Consciousness, Matter, and Miracles.* Santa Rosa, CA: Mountain of Love/Elite Books, 2005.

Myss, Caroline. *Anatomy of the Spirit: The Seven Stages of Power and Healing.* New York: Harmony Books, 1996.

Pert, Candace B., PhD. *Molecules of Emotion: The Science Behind Mind-Body Medicine.* New York: Simon & Schuster, 1999.

Schwartz, Gary E. *The Energy Healing Experiments: Science Reveals Our Natural Power to Heal.* New York: Atria Books, 2008.

Siegel, Bernie S., MD. *Love, Medicine & Miracles: Lessons Learned about Self-Healing from a Surgeon's Experience with Exceptional Patients.* New York: William Morrow Paperbacks, 1998.

### Websites

Association for Comprehensive Energy Psychology, www.energypsych.org

Donna Eden's website, www.innersource.net

EFT Universe, www.eftuniverse.com

Gary Craig's website, www.emofree.com

*To learn about Lyme disease, please visit the International Lyme and Associated Diseases Society, www.ilads.org, and consider taking part in the Lyme Disease Challenge, www.lymediseasechallenge.org.

## To Write to the Author

If you wish to contact the author or would like more information about this book, please write to the author in care of Llewellyn Worldwide Ltd. and we will forward your request. Both the author and publisher appreciate hearing from you and learning of your enjoyment of this book and how it has helped you. Llewellyn Worldwide Ltd. cannot guarantee that every letter written to the author can be answered, but all will be forwarded. Please write to:

Amy B. Scher
℅ Llewellyn Worldwide
2143 Wooddale Drive)
Woodbury, MN 55125-2989

Please enclose a self-addressed stamped envelope for reply,
or $1.00 to cover costs. If outside the U.S.A., enclose
an international postal reply coupon.

Many of Llewellyn's authors have websites with additional information and resources. For more information, please visit our website at http://www.llewellyn.com.